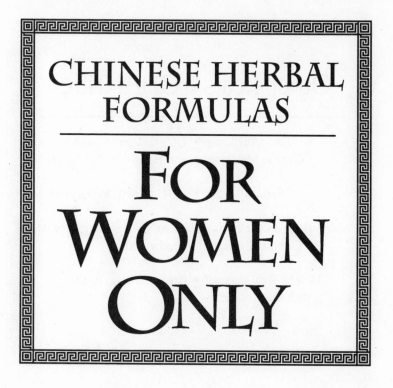

CHINESE HERBAL FORMULAS

FOR

WOMEN ONLY

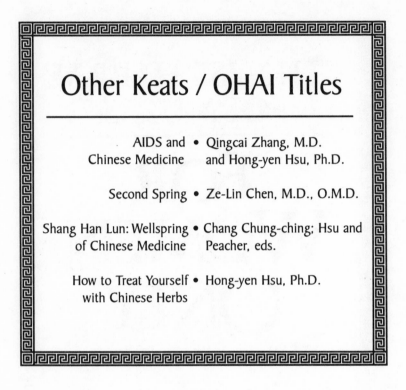

Other Keats / OHAI Titles

AIDS and • Qingcai Zhang, M.D.
Chinese Medicine   and Hong-yen Hsu, Ph.D.

Second Spring • Ze-Lin Chen, M.D., O.M.D.

Shang Han Lun: Wellspring • Chang Chung-ching; Hsu and
of Chinese Medicine   Peacher, eds.

How to Treat Yourself • Hong-yen Hsu, Ph.D.
with Chinese Herbs

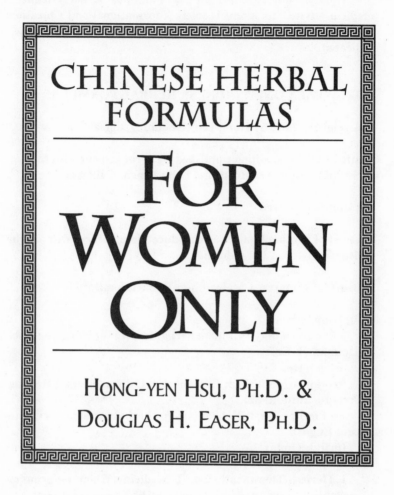

CHINESE HERBAL FORMULAS

FOR WOMEN ONLY

HONG-YEN HSU, PH.D. &
DOUGLAS H. EASER, PH.D.

Keats Publishing, Inc. ✖ New Canaan, Connecticut
Oriental Healing Arts Institute ⏀ Long Beach, California

For Women Only: Chinese Herbal Formulas is not intended as medical advice. Its intent is solely informational and educational. Please consult a health professional should the need for one be indicated.

FOR WOMEN ONLY: CHINESE HERBAL FORMULAS

Copyright © 1982 by Hong-yen Hsu and Douglas H. Easer

Keats Publishing edition published by arrangement with the Oriental Healing Arts Institute, Long Beach, California.

Library of Congress Cataloging-in-Publication Data

Hsü, Hung-yüan.
    For women only : Chinese herbal formulas / Hong-yen Hsu, Douglas H. Easer.
        p. cm.
    Previously published: Los Angeles, Calif. : Oriental Healing Arts Institute, 1982.
    Text in English, with headings for herbal formulas in Chinese and English.
    Includes index.
    ISBN 0-87983-654-7
    1. Herbs—Therapeutic use. 2. Medicine, Chinese-Formulae, receipts, prescriptions. 3. Women—Diseases—Treatment. 4. Women—Health and hygiene. I. Easer, Douglas H. II. Title.
    RM666.H33H78 1995
    615'.321'082—dc20   95-2505
                                                                   CIP

Printed in the United States of America

Published by Keats Publishing, Inc.
27 Pine Street (Box 876)
New Canaan, Connecticut 06840-0876

98 97 96 95 6 5 4 3 2 1

Table of Contents

Notice

The following is a summary description of some of the natural herbal formulas widely used throughout Asia. The information compiled from traditional medical texts and from the observations of modern authorities on Chinese medicine is presented here for its educational value and should not be used for diagnosis, treatment, or prevention of disease without the advice of a Chinese physician or other medical authority.

Preface

In China and Southeast Asia, medical problems are treated by Western as well as traditional Chinese therapies. Although both systems share a common goal, the alleviation of pain and prolongation of life, they differ considerably in theory and practice. Western medicine focuses on identification of cause and specific treatment. Medicine in general is not prescribed if the cause is unknown or undecided. In contrast, the Chinese doctor does not need to identify the illness in modern medical terms. Rather, he assesses the patient's subjective complaints, or conformation, and prescribes a holistic treatment. In short, modern medicine relies on accurate diagnosis of the disease and its cause while Chinese medicine focuses on the patient's reactions, subjective and objective, and treats disease as unique to the individual.

Western medicine has undoubtably made great strides in the diagnosis and treatment of disease. However, its therapeutic approach has its limitations. Such disorders as hepatitis, diabetes mellitus, nephrosis, heart disease, rheumatism, hypertension, arteriosclerosis, allergies, women's psychosomatic problems, and cancer have proven virtually impervious to treatment with Western medicine. Surprisingly they are more effectively dealt with by Chinese medicine.

Most Western drugs are synthetic analogues of natural substances. In many cases, these drugs upon introduction have seemingly miraculous effects against certain diseases.

However, after awhile, due to their high toxicity, their side effects grow more apparent. All too obvious examples are penicillin anaphylaxis, thalidomide teratogenicity, and the adverse effects of corticosteroids. These deleterious side effects necessitate a re-evaluation of Western medicine.

On the other hand, Chinese medicine uses natural substances almost entirely, and medicinals which are very potent and highly poisonous constitute only a small part of the Chinese pharmacopeia. On the average, the toxicity of most Chinese herbs is very minute. Chinese medicine has been used successfully for thousands of years.

About ten years ago, I inventoried Chinese herb physicians and herbal pharmacies in order to determine what type of patient was most frequently seen and what formulas were most frequently prescribed. I found that women with gynecological problems visited doctors most frequently, and the most frequently prescribed formulas were for gynecological and non-surgical conditions. These conclusions are based on visits to 10 percent of the 3000 herbal physicians practicing in Taiwan, as well as visits to 1,000 herbal pharmacies out of a total of 7,000.

It is customary for most Oriental women to see an herb doctor for gynecological disorders because Western medicine is unable to make a conclusive diagnosis of and provide effective treatment for such frequent irritating complaints as headache, insomnia, neurotic behavior, psychosomatic disorders, vertigo, tinnitus, lumbago, palpitations, and chills. Chinese medicine is uniquely suited to treating these disorders.

Why is it that Chinese medicine can treat illnesses that Western medicine cannot? Essentially Chinese medicine has developed a theoretic framework that Western medicine lacks. One principle is, maintain the body in a well-balanced state; supplement weakness and purge firmness. In addition, "blood," "water," and "ch'i," theories are not found in Western medicine. The three theories are briefly stated below.

1. Blood. Chinese medicine holds that if menstrual

blood or the blood of childbirth is not expelled it accumulates in the body, causing obstruction to the flow of blood, fiuid, and *ch'i*. This condition is known as blood stagnation. In a young person such a condition will probably go unnoticed until they reach forty or fifty years of age when it causes vertigo, lumbago, palpitations, and so on. Chinese medicine easily treats disorders attributed to blood stagnation. Herbs such as *tang-kuei* and cnidium are used for this purpose.

2. Water. If water is not excreted it accumulates in the body and such symptoms such as edema, arthritis, oliguria, or polyuria appear. For water stagnation herbs such as hoelen, polyporus and alisma promote diuresis.

3. *Ch'i.* *Ch'i* in relation to the body is vitality or "physiological energy." *Ch'i* can be static and mobile. Mobile *ch'i* means *ch'i* is up-rushing causing dizziness, headache, and "flushing," or what the Japanese call "nobose." Static *ch'i* means *ch'i* is obstructed and accumulated in one place instead of flowing. Diseases of *ch'i* cannot be found with X-ray machines, sophisticated instruments, or biochemical examination but recent research provides scientific verification of its existence. Magnolia bark and perilla are effective in treating *ch'i* problems. These theories are discussed in greater detail in the text.

I am very grateful to the staff of the Oriental Healing Arts Institute for their efforts in compiling this book. Douglas H. Easer translated the introduction and collated the herbal formulas. Nancy Hays researched, wrote, and edited the sections on Western medicine, and Judith Haueter edited the final version. I am also grateful to Ms. Wang Shu-kuei for proofreading the manuscript.

Hong-yen Hsu, Ph.D
July 1, 1981

ix

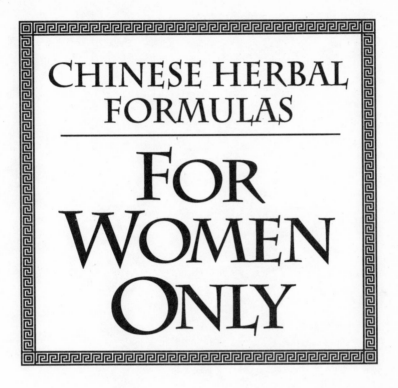

CHINESE HERBAL FORMULAS

FOR WOMEN ONLY

Introduction

When a Western doctor cannot discover a physiological cause for an illness, he usually concludes that the illness is mental and recommends psychiatric treatment. The Chinese doctor approaches illness in a completely different manner. In Chinese medicine the cause of an illness is secondary—treatment focuses on the "conformation" of the symptoms presented. In a sense, a Chinese doctor follows the axiom that the whole is greater than the sum of the parts. For instance, an illness usually begins in one part of the body, but sooner or later it affects the rest of the body. Western medicine generally concerns itself with the locus of the disease whereas Chinese medicine adopts a holistic approach and treats all the symptoms as a unit. Medication made of natural rather than synthetic substances is administered according to the conformation--all the symptoms, mental and physical, objective and subjective. To further delineate the two, the chart below compares modern and Chinese medicine.

Modern Medicine	Chinese Medicine
1. Mechanistic theory of disease based on scientific study	1. Philosophic theory based on empirical evidence
2. Partial body treatment	2. Whole body treatment

3. Diagnosis based on objective factors	3. Diagnosis based on subjective as well as objective factors
4. Synthetic or chemical drugs	4. Natural nutritive drugs
5. Ineffective therapy for many chronic diseases	5. Very effective therapy for chronic ailments

For the benefit of our Western readers, a brief overview of Chinese medicine and Chinese medicine in relation to gynecological problems follows.

Ch'i Diseases

Of vital importance to diagnosis in Chinese medicine is the state of the patient's *ch'i*. The term *ch'i* has no equivalent in English. It has been variously translated as "air," "breath," "vitality," or "bio-energy"--in other words, the life force. *Ch'i*, mobile and without form, flows through the body like blood and water (fluid), circulating through and along the acupuncture meridians. *Ch'i* diseases affect the nervous system, the meridians, and ultimately the mind and spirit. *Ch'i* conformations stem from the "seven emotions," and are treated the same as other illnesses--with herbal medicines. Dr. Gonzan Goto, a Japanese authority on Chinese medicine, goes so far as to contend that the obstruction of *ch'i* causes all disease. In contrast, with no concept of *ch'i*, modern medicine treats emotional illness as a separate problem even though the victim is suffering physically.

One type of *ch'i* illness is called "ascending *ch'i*." The afflicted have opposing symptoms of extremely cold hands and feet and a hot, flushed face. It is believed that *ch'i* is now trapped in the upper body. (The Japanese call this condition *nobose*.) *Cinnamomium cassia* treats ascending *ch'i* by normalizing and regulating its flow. Note: Cinnamon by itself is too weak and needs to be taken in combination with other herbs for maximum effect.

2

Ch'i stagnated in the lower portion of the body is called "obstructed *ch'i*." The main subjective symptom is the sensation that a foreign object is stuck in the throat. Other symptoms are chest discomfort, shortness of breath, and palpitations to the extent that the heart is pounding and the person feels that it is going to stop beating altogether. Obstructed *ch'i* also causes disorder of the pulse, meaning an irregular pulse that intermittently stops. The most effective herbs for obstructed *ch'i* are magnolia bark (*hou-pu*) and perilla (*tzu-su-yeh*), or perilla fruit (*tzu-su-tzu*), and the best formula, Pinellia and Magnolia Combination (*Pan-hsia-hou-pu-tang*).

The Seven Emotions

The origins of *ch'i* diseases are very hard to diagnose. People with no serious physical symptoms may suffer from these diseases along with those who display symptoms of every type of degenerative condition.

However, since *ch'i* diseases are inextricably linked to the seven emotions, it seems appropriate to discuss them. According to Chinese medical theory, diseases are brought about by either external or internal causes. External causes are due mainly to climate and environment and are called the "six excesses", namely, wind, dryness, cold, fire, moisture, and heat. Internal causes are the "seven emotions", namely, pleasure, anger, anxiety, pensiveness or brooding, sorrow or grief, fear, and shock or terror. Excessive emotional stimulation or inhibition causes imbalances which eventually injure the viscera. Conformations resulting from the seven emotions are mainly diseases of *ch'i* but the blood can be affected too. As was said before, *ch'i* diseases affect the nervous system, the acupuncture meridian system, the blood, and the mind. Such diverse conditions as schizophrenia and Parkinson's disease are included in this category.

Anger stimulates *ch'i*, pleasure calms *ch'i*, anxiety obstructs *ch'i*, brooding coagulates *ch'i*, grief reduces *ch'i*, fear suppresses *ch'i*, and shock disturbs *ch'i*. Further, anger by stimulating *ch'i* injures the liver and extreme anger causes the blood to congest in the upper torso. Characterized by a ruddy face and red eyes, this reaction can bring on a coma and sudden apoplexy. Since the liver controls mood, the principle of treatment is to inhibit, clean, and nourish the liver. One formula used for this is the *Tang-kuei* and Bupleurum Formula (*Hsiao-yao-san*) and Bupleurum Formula (*I-kan-san*). (*I-kan-san* literally means "angry liver formula.")

Extreme, continual pleasure calms *ch'i* but in so doing injures the heart. The patient becomes manic and mental illness ensues. In addition, according to Chinese medical science, the seven emotions closely interrelate with the five elements, namely, metal, wood, water, fire, and earth. Mutually interlinked, the five elements reciprocally produce and destroy each other. Since the heart corresponds to fire, and fire to pleasure, the principle of treatment is to purge and nourish or tone up the heart. One of the formulas used is Coptis and Scute Combination (*Huang-lien-chieh-tu-tang*).

Grief weakens *ch'i* and injures the lungs; its outward manifestations are facial pallor, depression, and sadness. If grief persists, the patient becomes neurotic and eventually pyschotic. Grief corresponds to metal and the principle of treatment is to tone up the lungs. The herbal formula often used is the Platycodon and Fritillary Combination (*Ching-fei-tang*).

Brooding coagulates *ch'i* and injures the spleen. This results in a lack of appetite, a condition often seen in children. Brooding belongs to the earth. Treatment strengthens the spleen with such herbal formulas as Hoelen Five Herb Formula (*Wu-ling-san*) and Ginseng and Atractylodes Formula (*Sheng-ling-pai-chu-san*).

Shock is triggered by external stimuli and disturbs *ch'i* while fear originates within and suppresses *ch'i*. Both injure the kidneys. Severe injury to the kidneys causes mental disorders. Malfunctioning kidneys are also linked to sexual disorders and diabetes. Fright, or shock, and fear belong to water. The principle of treatment is to nourish the kidneys and fortify the sperm. One of the most versatile supple-

4

menting and nourishing formulas is Rehmannia Eight Formula (*Pá-wei-ti-huang-wan*).

Anxiety obstructs *ch'i* which in turn injures the lungs as well as the spleen. Depression, sullenness, and loss of appetite are the obvious manifestations.

Chinese medicine also believes that the relative weakness or firmness of the five solid viscera instigate emotional changes, a concept not found in Western medicine. In other words, an appraisal of the mental-emotional state can help determine the condition of the viscera and hence dictate the appropriate herbal therapy. Although modern medicine includes psychoanalysis and recognizes the interaction between mind and body, it lacks the encompassing methods developed by Chinese medical theory to treat disease resulting from this interaction. Another way to look at the different approaches is to compare basic cultural philosophy. An Occidental generally looks at life in a linear, Aristotelean mode, separating large groups into smaller ones and assigning cause and effect to events. The Oriental, on the other hand, views life as circular or spherical and events as constant interactions without specific causes and effects or beginnings and endings. The two cultures' medical theories basically reflect their life views, one being scientific and the other philosophical.

Water Diseases

Many diseases are caused by disturbances in water metabolism--an imbalance in the circulation of the body fluids or abnormal distribution of water throughout the body. Chinese herbal medicine calls water stagnation within the stomach *"tan yin"* (sputum drink). Fluid stagnation in the bronchi is called *"chih yin"* (branch drink), and renal edema is called *"yi yin"* (overflow drink). Water stagnation is indicated by kidney disorders; puffiness in the face; heart disease; edema of the lower parts of the body, legs, and feet; pleurisy; and stomach weakness accompanied by gurgling sounds. Symptoms of water intoxication, many of which can be directly observed, are vertigo; a ringing sound in the ears; headache; excessive or diminished sweating or its complete absence (anhidrosis); excessive mucus; rheumatism; frequent or infrequent urination; pounding heart; and a heavy head.

Western medicine calls the action of increasing excretion of urine "diuresis" while Chinese medicine refers to it as "water delivery." Western medicine uses a variety of diuretics, but many of them have pronounced side effects. Chinese medicine also uses many water delivering herbs in treatment, such as polyporus, hoelen, alisma, akebia, *ma-huang,* and atractylodes. These herbs tend to be gentle acting and effectively treat chronic nephritis and uremia, illnesses which Western medicine regards as recalcitrant. Formulas are Hoelen Five Herb Formula, Polyporus Combination, and Ginger and Hoelen Combination. Incidentally, according to clinical experience, blood, water, and *ch'i* illnesses do not occur singly but in combination.

Chill Diseases

Anemia, edema coupled with the congestion of blood in a part, hyperemia, and water intoxication bring about chill symptoms. Other factors are air-conditioning, flushing reaction, and moderate fevers in the limbs. Chilling commonly accompanies gynecological problems, but it stands to reason that men too are subject to it. However, the typical patient is usually of a weak conformation, a conformation more common in women. Also, due to their menses, women are more subject to blood congestion and anemia, and chilling is a by-product of these conditions. Chilling can be cured within a week with the Aconite and G.L. Combination (*Szu-ni-tang*). Aconite and G.L. Combination contains licorice, dried ginger, and aconite. (Aconite is toxic if taken in large amounts, but Chinese pharmacists have long known how to reduce its

6

toxicity.) *Tang-kuei,* Evodia, and Ginger Combination, another definitive formula for chill disorders, treats people of weak conformation. The indications are poor physical condition, facial pallor, easy fatigability, and cold extremities. *Tang-kuei,* Evodia, and Ginger Combination is also good for frigorism and stomatitis.

Blood Diseases

Blood disease includes all conditions associated with malfunctions of the circulatory system: "blood stagnation," anemia, varicose veins, hardening of the arteries, and hemorrhages. Blood stagnation is a theory exclusive to Chinese medicine. In modern medicine it resembles "extravasated blood" in which blood passes out of its proper place as when a vessel ruptures. The traditional Chinese view looked upon stagnant or stagnated blood as "filthy blood other than that from menstruation." Later on it came to mean "blocked" instead of "filthy." The term first appeared in *The Yellow Emperor's Classic of Internal Medicine* (Nei ching) and later in the *Treatise on Febrile Diseases* (Shang han lun) and *Summaries of Household Remedies* (Chin kuei yao lueh). The causes of stagnant blood incorporate the following factors: (1) heredity, (2) menopause and childbirth, (3) gynecological diseases, (4) fevers, (5) circulatory disorders, (6) liver disorders, (7) chronic inflammation, (8) excessive lipids, (9) hormonal imbalance, and (10) food poisoning. A series of studies by Dr. M. H. Knisely at the University of Chicago in the 1940s tends to corroborate the theory of stagnated blood. He used the term "sludged blood" meaning the coagulation of red blood cells in blood vessels. The blood stagnation theory has enabled Chinese medicine to create many effective therapeutic methods not found in modern medicine for coping with chronic diseases.

Acute lower abdominal pain is a primary symptom of blood stagnation. When diagnosing, the doctor asks the patient to lie down on his or her back with legs outstretched. The doctor then quickly and lightly palpates the left side of the lower abdomen, using his index, middle, and ring fingers. If there is blood stagnation, the patient will feel intense pain when the area is palpated and will respond immediately by bending his knees. This condition seldom occurs on the right side and patients with these symptoms are usually women. The Persica and Rhubarb Combination (*Tao-ho-cheng-chi-tang*) is frequently used for treatment.

Gynecological Diseases

About 70 percent of a Chinese doctor's patients are women because they are more prone to blood and *ch'i* diseases. The special health matters relating to a woman's reproductive system belong to the branch of medicine known as gynecology. For example, among the health concerns specific to women are menstrual disorders. When a woman's menstrual pattern varies noticeably from the usual one, in the absence of pregnancy, it signals a physical or emotional disorder. Generally, Chinese medicine regards menstrual and other gynecological problems as blood disease. Usually these blood disorders result from "blood stagnation" which most often occurs in women due to the physiological consequences of menstruation and childbirth. Blood stagnation in women involves non-menstrual blood poisoned by bacteria and, in some cases, external injury.

Chinese medicine classifies the following disorders as gynecological when occurring in women.

1. Fatigue
2. Shoulder stiffness
3. Headache
4. Insomnia
5. Menopausal disorders
6. Neurosis
7. Chill conformation
8. *Nobose* (ascending *ch'i* which causes flushing up)

9. Dizziness
10. Tinnitus
11. Lower abdominal pain
12. Pain in the waist
13. Gastric dilation
14. Hysteria
15. Menstrual aberrations
16. Painful menstruation
17. Excessive bleeding
18. Leukorrhea
19. Illness during pregnancy, postpartum illness
20. Maculae
21. Constipation
22. Anemia
23. High and low blood pressure
24. Abdominal puffiness

Numbers 15, 16, 17, 18, 19, 20, 22, 23, 24 belong to the category of gynecological disorders. Numbers 1 through 14 are symptoms associated with gynecological problems.

Many gynecological disorders, as mentioned previously, are caused by *ch'i*. The clinical symptoms of *ch'i* diseases follow.

Whole Body Diseases

1. Exhaustion: easily fatigued, loss of and decreased sexual desire
2. Insomnia: easily aroused from sleep—light sleeper; frequent dreaming—dreaming about eating
3. *Nobose:* blood stagnation, red face, headache, heavy head, blurred vision, ringing in the ears, obstructed vision, throat discomfort, hoarseness, cough without sound, throat obstruction
4. Profuse sweating over the whole body or in a portion thereof
5. Stiff shoulders and neck, sore waist and back
6. Muscular pain in whole body or portion thereof; nervousness
7. Chest discomfort: shortness of breath, palpitations,

pounding heart, a feeling that the heart is going to stop
8. Pulse disorder (*bu-cheng-mai*): very slow or quick pulse, or irregular pulse which sometimes stops
9. Discomfort in the stomach and intestines: no appetite, nausea, vomiting, thirst, disordered taste and smell
10. The entire body or a part of it feels warm; a chill sensation; nausea; paralysis; painful itching; sensitivity; paralysis
11. Frequent urination, painful urination, urination during the night, constipation, diarrhea, irregular menstruation, chill disorders

Nerve Disorders
1. Not feeling well upon awakening in the morning
2. Pessimistic, melancholic
3. Lack of interest, no interest in reading or watching television
4. Inability to concentrate, inattentive listener
5. Lassitude, poor worker
6. Dizziness, easily fatigued
7. Diminished ability to think and remember (diminished memory)
8. Indecision
9. Anxiety, irritability
10. Insecurity
11. Self-reproach
12. Despair
13. Overly reflective
14. Aversion to seeing people: self-isolation, highly critical rather than complimentary
15. Constantly doing work that has already been done
16. Mysophobia: insistence on cleanliness
17. Self-destructive urge: urge to commit suicide, urge to kill others
18. Feels faint at a certain stage of illness; emotionless, expressionless, taciturn

Upon first contracting a chronic condition, a patient's

family is sympathetic, but concern diminishes as the condition persists. The stress within the family then aggravates the symptoms. If Chinese medicine can relieve the vicious cycle, it should be a welcome addition to Western treatment. As said before, Chinese medicine classifies all female disorders as diseases of the blood and *ch'i* and as such the blood and *ch'i* are the objects of treatment.

Stagnant blood means that the blood contains toxins, but also that the passage of blood is obstructed by some hardness causing poor circulation. A change in the rate of blood circulation gives rise to "blood stagnation." In addition to lower abdominal pain, the symptoms are a heavy head, itchy scalp, shoulder stiffness, dizziness, tinnitus, and a dry mouth. Furthermore, the abdomen feels full but actually is not; the body or a portion thereof feels feverish; the skin and mucous membranes have red spots; the blood vessels are swollen; goose pimples appear on the skin; the skin is excessively dry; the edges of the tongue turn dark purple and the lips pale; and the gums turn dark red or blue and bleed easily. There are feelings of chills at the waist and numbness, plus insomnia, amnesia, and constipation. Stagnant blood-dispelling medicine is required to treat these symptoms. For a yang conformation raw herbs such as apricot seeds, moutan, and paeonia are used. Typical formulas are Persica and Rhubarb Combination (*Tao-ho-cheng-chi-tang*) and Cinnamon and Hoelen Formula (*Kuei-chih-fu-ling-wan*). A weak conformation accompanied by blood stagnation calls for *tang-kuei*, and *Cnidium officinale* Makino (cnidium) which is the *Tang-kuei* Four Combination (*Szu-wu-tang*). In persistent cases of blood stagnation the Chinese rely on such animal drugs as leeches and gadflies.

Chinese medicine uses the formulas mentioned above to treat the following disorders: abnormal menstruation, *hsieh chih tao*[1], pregnancy problems, postpartum problems,

---

[1] A professor at Fukushima University using modern medical methods noted that the *hsieh chih tao* conformation is a disorder of the autonomic nervous system found only in menopausal women. A former chairman of the Oriental Medicine Association also studied the phenomenon and concluded that it is linked to the biological makeup of women and injuries to the nervous system.

11

obstruction of blood circulation, artēriosclerosis, and uterine bleeding. A normal, healthy woman experiences menstruation, pregnancy, childbirth, and menopause. If her biological makeup is abnormal, however, she might have successive spontaneous abortions or miscarriages and develop blood stagnancy which in turn causes neurosis, or mental problems, and menstrual irregularity and aberrations. Blood stagnation injures the autonomic nervous system. Its symptoms are leukorrhea, bleeding, and menstrual disorders.

For ease in reading, this book has been arranged in the form of a manual. In this way the reader can peruse the entire text or merely read those sections of interest to him or her. Because it has been written in this manner, however, a certain amount of repetition of material was necessary. First the disease or disorder is described in Western terms. Then the appropriate Chinese formulas for the condition are listed. Since Chinese formulas are wide-spectrum treatments, many combinations appear under several categories.

Chinese herbal therapy is analogous to megavitamin therapy in that it aims at correcting body imbalances while simultaneously building healthier tissues and blood. We hope the following discussion of gynecological problems further reveals the multifaceted nature of Chinese medicine.

GYNECOLOGICAL PROBLEMS

1. Endometritis

The vitally important endometrium lines the uterus and as such is the site of implantation of a fertilized ovum. Endometritis is the inflammation of the endometrium and neck of the uterus caused by the growth of suppurative bacteria. Poor hygiene during and after intercourse, childbirth, abortion, menstruation, uterine curettage, probe insertion, or carelessly inserted forceps introduce the bacteria to this fertile breeding ground. Frequently implicated are gonococcus, Mycobacterium tuberculosis, *Escherichia coli*, staphylococcus, and streptococcus bacilli. An irregular diet and lifestyle, malposition of the uterus, tumors, a retained placenta, lead poisoning, and blood disorders also make the uterus highly susceptible to infection. In severe cases infection spreads to the uterine wall.

Women who want to bear children must be alert to the presence of endometritis because it can cause habitual abortion or even sterility. Since the infection easily becomes chronic, it must be treated as quickly as possible. Other terms used interchangeably with endometritis are substantial inflammation and peripheral inflammation of the uterus.

13

Symptoms

Discomfort or pain in the lower abdomen; malodorous, milky or yellow leukorrhea (discharge from the cervical canal or vagina) consisting of mucus and pus, and sometimes blood; painful menstruation (dysmenorrhea); bleeding during intercourse; vaginal inflammation; itching around the vagina; chills; fever; irritability; and loss of appetite.

Treatment

Early diagnosis and treatment are important and should be sought when the first symptoms of discomfort and leukorrhea appear. Women past menopause are particularly vulnerable to chronic infection because the endometrium no longer regenerates during the course of a menstrual cycle. Endometritis easily becomes chronic and results in many complications if not immediately and completely eradicated. Household remedies do not cure endometritis. Antibiotics are prescribed for acute inflammations. Chinese herb formulas are effective for chronic inflammations. Note: Endometritis can be very serious and proper treatment often requires hospitalization and intravenous antibiotics.

Chinese Herbal Formulas

Gentiana Combination
(*Lung-tan-hsieh-kan-tang*) 龍膽瀉肝湯

First recorded in the Chinese medical work *Hsueh-shih i an* by Hsueh Chi of the Ming dynasty.

Herbal Components

5.0g *tang-kuei*	1.0g gardenia	1.0g licorice
5.0g rehmannia	5.0g akebia	1.0g gentiana
3.0g scute	3.0g plantago	3.0g alisma

Indications

Pain in the armpits, deafness, swollen ears, blood in the urine, gonorrhea, swelling and itching in the genital area, leukorrhea, coated yellow tongue, strong pulse, tense abdominal tendons, resistant pain when pressed on the lower abdomen along the *kan* (liver) meridian, and redness of the mouth, tongue, and eyes.

Uses

Strong conformations with moisture heat of the *kan* (liver) meridian and acute or chronic endometritis due to bacterial infection. Also leukorrhea as a complication of urethritis and cystitis. Generally, smilax (3g) and coix (5g) are added.

Cinnamon and Hoelen Formula
(*Kuei-chih-fu-ling-wan*) 桂枝茯苓丸

First recorded in the Chinese medical work *Summaries of Household Remedies* (Chin kuei yao lueh A.D. 205) as a treatment for gynecological disorders involving stagnant blood and also as a drug for men.

Herbal Components

| 4.0g cinnamon | 4.0g moutan | 4.0g paeonia |
| 4.0g hoelen | 4.0g persica | |

Cinnamon checks flushing up of blood and coordinates the effects of the other herbs on blood circulation. Hoelen with cinnamon cures abdominal palpitations and is a diuretic. Persica removes stagnant blood and increases blood circulation. Moutan removes stagnant blood and increases vitality. Paeonia expels stagnant blood.

15

Indications

Strong constitution with a flushed face, protruding abdomen, resistant pressing pain at the umbilicus, tense and sunken pulse, headache, shoulder stiffness, vertigo, and chills in the feet.

Uses

Strong conformations with endometritis due to retained placenta; myoma of the uterus with leukorrhea; abdominal pain; a sensation of heavy pressure at the lower abdomen; and excessive or difficult menstruation. For constipation, rhubarb (1.5 - 2.0g) is added.

*Persica and Rhubarb Combination
(*Tao-ho-cheng-chi-tang*) 桃核承氣湯

Herbal Components

5.0g persica	4.0g cinnamon	1.5g licorice
3.0g rhubarb	2.0g mirabilitum	

Persica and cinnamon dispel stagnant blood in the lower abdomen and improve blood circulation. Cinnamon in combination with licorice relieves flushing up. Rhubarb and mirabilitum dispel "internal heat."

Indications

Noticeable resistance and pain in lower abdomen when pressed.

Uses

Serious endometritis.

The symbol* means that a herbal formula has been approved for use in medical facilities by the Department of Pharmaceutical Affairs, Ministry of Health and Welfare, Japan.

*Rhubarb and Moutan Combination
(*Ta-huang-mu-tan-pi-tang*) 大黃牡丹皮湯

Herbal Components
  2.0g rhubarb 6.0g benincasa 4.0g persica
  4.0g moutan   4.0g mirabilitum
Rhubarb and mirabilitum, the major components in this
formula, dispel "internal heat" and relieve inflammation.
Benincasa is an antipyretic. Moutan is an antipyretic and
refrigerant that dispels stagnant blood. Persica dispels stagnant blood and "internal heat."

Indications
  Copious, malodorous leukorrhea with pus; pain and
fullness at the lower abdomen; and severe pain during
urination.

Uses
  Serious endometritis, urethritis, cystitis, and pelvic
congestion.

Tang-kuei and Eight Herb Formula
(*Pa-wei-tai-hsia-fang*) 八味帶下方

A commonly used formula from *Min chia fang hsuan* by
Mototsune Yamada of Japan.

Herbal Components
  4.0g smilax 3.0g akebia 1.0g lonicera
  5.0g *tang-kuei* 3.0g hoelen 1.0g rhubarb
  3.0g cnidium 2.0g citrus
Smilax and lonicera detoxify and dispel internal heat.
Tang-kuei and cnidium nourish the blood. Hoelen, akebia,
and citrus dispel moist heat and water toxin.

17

Indications

Leukorrhea (discharge from the female genital canal) with moist heat, mild anemia, subacute inflammation, and congestion.

Uses

Subacute or chronic endometritis with yellow or white leukorrhea. If there is no constipation, rhubarb may be omitted.

*Tang-kuei and Paeonia Formula (Tang-kuei-shao-yao-san) 當歸芍藥散

First mentioned in the ancient Chinese medical work *Summaries of Household Remedies* (Chin kuei yao lueh A.D. 205) of the Han dynasty.

Herbal Components

3.0g *tang-kuei*   4.0g paeonia   4.0g atractylodes
3.0g cnidium   4.0g hoelen   4.0g alisma

Tang-kuei, a hematinic and nutritive, synthesizes the actions of the herbs and eases pain. Atractylodes is a diuretic. Cnidium increases vitality and nourishes the blood. Hoelen dispels inner fluid accumulation and is compatible with atractylodes and alisma.

Uses

Weak conformations without inflammation but with congestion, mild anemia, chills, and a tendency towards fatigue; leukorrhea due to chronic endometritis; frequent urination and abdominal pus; low back pain.

*Bupleurum and Paeonia Formula
(*Chia-wei-hsiao-yao-san*) 加味逍遙散

Both the medical dictionary of the Sung dynasty, *Tai ping huei min ho chi chu fang* (A.D. 1110), and the *Standards for Treatment* (Cheng chih chun sheng A.D. 1602) of the Ming dynasty list Bupleurum and Paeonia Formula for gynecological problems.

The *Japanese Medical News* No. 1837 also reports that this formula is the best basic remedy for cirrhosis and very effective for abdominal tension; thirst; persistent, bitter taste in the mouth; headache; turbid urine; nosebleeds; and odontorrhagia.

Herbal Components

3.0g *tang-kuei*	3.0g paeonia	3.0g atractylodes
3.0g hoelen	3.0g bupleurum	2.0g licorice
2.0g moutan	2.0g gardenia	1.0g ginger
1.0g mentha		

The principal herbs of this formula are *tang-kuei*, paeonia, and bupleurum. *Tang-kuei* is a mild agent for dispelling extravasated blood and a hematinic. Paeonia, a mild anticonvulsant and analgesic agent, and *tang-kuei* have been used for blood diseases for 2,000 years. Bupleurum is an antipyretic-stomachic agent for chest distention with resistance and pain when pressed and alternating chills and fever. It is a principal herb for liver ailments. Gardenia, which is antiphlogistic, analgesic, and hemastatic, is given for depression, a "glowing" feeling, jaundice, anxiety, and insomnia. Moutan, a sedative and anticonvulsive, is given for headache and low back pain; it also may be used for hypertension, inflammation, bleeding, stagnant blood, and gynecopathy. Atractylodes and hoelen are stomachics and diuretics. Mentha is cooling, antidepressive, and a stomachic.

Indications

Aching in the arms and legs, dizziness, mental instability, flushing, thirst, night sweating with fever, anorexia, narcolepsy or insomnia, cardiac and limb fever, earache, abdominal distention near the umbilicus, turbid or residual urine, hot flashes, menstrual irregularity.

Uses

The semi-strong and semi-weak type; chronic and weak conformation with a disorder of the autonomic nervous system, menstrual aberration, abdominal pain, leukorrhea, and stagnant blood. Also obvious neurotic symptoms which accompany stagnant blood, such as fever and chills, fever in the limbs, heaviness of the head, vertigo, ruddy face, night sweats, insomnia, generalized tiredness, and loss of appetite.

*Tang-kuei and Gelatin Combination (Chiung-kuei-chiao-ai-tang) 芎歸膠艾湯

First mentioned in the ancient Chinese medical text *Summaries of Household Remedies* (Chin kuei yao lueh A.D. 205) of the Han dynasty.

Herbal Components

4.0g *tang-kuei*	3.0g cnidium	4.0g paeonia
3.0g licorice	3.0g artemisia	5.0g rehmannia
3.0g gelatin	(mugwort)	

Cnidium dispels stagnant blood. Gelatin, licorice, *tang-kuei,* rehmannia, and paeonia are blood tonics that nourish the uterus. Artemisia is an astringent and hemostatic which also nourishes the uterus. Gelatin and artemisia are important components for preventing miscarriage.

Uses

Chronic conformation with leukorrhea, tendency towards anemia, frequent bleeding of the uterus, hot sensation in the limbs, spasms at the left side of the abdomen, weakness at the abdomen, and abdominal pain.

20

*Ginseng and Longan Combination
(*Kuei-pi-tang*) 歸脾湯

First recorded in *Life Preserving Prescriptions* (Chi sheng fang) by Yen Yung-ho of the Sung dynasty.

Herbal Components
3.0g ginseng	3.0g hoelen	1.0g polygala
2.0g astragalus	1.0g ginger	1.0g inula
3.0g longan	2.0g *tang-kuei*	1.0g licorice
3.0g atractylodes	1.0g jujube	3.0g zizyphus

Ginseng, astragalus, atractylodes, hoelen, jujube, and licorice nourish the spleen and stomach. Longan, polygala, and zizyphus seed are hematinics and sedatives. Inula cures mental instability. Ginger is a stomachic. *Tang-kuei* nourishes the blood.

Indications
Loss of appetite, nervousness, insomnia, amnesia.

2. Uterine Myoma

Myomas are tumors that contain muscle tissue. The most common myomas are those found on the myometrium (uterine wall). They are not malignant. Studies show about 25 percent of women develop myomas after the age of thirty-five. Although the growth of uterine myomas corresponds to the function of ovarian hormones, the basic cause has not yet been found. A myoma at the neck of the uterus or cervix presses on the bladder and rectum. A myoma beneath the mucous membrane causes endometritis; delayed, painful, and excessive menstruation; and severe, postpartum bleeding if present at delivery. Sometimes the myoma delivers itself through the cervix; this is called "parturition from myoma." Myomas range in size from that of a finger to that of a child's head.

Symptoms

Tiny myomas have no apparent symptoms, but large myomas put pressure on the rectum and bladder causing constipation or blockage. Uterine myomas may cause irregular bleeding or excessive menstruation, and some women have low back pain or a cold sensation around the waist. Young women become aware of myomas after an abortion or during and after childbirth because of excessive bleeding. Massive hemorrhaging induces anemia, palpitations, gasping, and a rapid pulse.

Treatment

Women who fear that a myoma is a latent cancer should be reassured that uterine myomas are completely different from malignant tumors and do not become cancerous. Small myomas which show no signs of growth do not require surgery or other treatment but should be kept under observation through regular physical examinations. Sometimes anti-extravasated blood agents dissolve egg-sized tumors, but in severe cases which have been treated for several months without improvement, surgery is required.

Chinese Herbal Formulas

Chinese herb formulas cannot cure uterine myomas. However, they can alleviate the uncomfortable symptoms that accompany premenopausal uterine myomas of moderate size.

*Tang-kuei and Gelatin Combination
(*Chiung-kuei-chiao-ai-tang*) 芎歸膠艾湯

See page 20.

Indications
Bleeding, anemia, a sensation of pressure in the lower abdomen, pain during intercourse.

*Persica and Rhubarb Combination
(*Tao-ho-cheng-chi-tang*) 桃核承氣湯

See page 16.

Indications
Noticeable resistance and pain when pressed on the lower abdomen.

Uses
Stagnant blood; serious endometritis caused by myomas.

3. Uterine Cancer

A carcinoma is a malignant tumor that tends to spread. The incidence of uterine cancer roughly equals that of stomach cancer in women. Tumors grow either in the endometrial wall or the cervix. Younger women more commonly develop cervical carcinoma and older women (forty to sixty years of age), endometrial carcinoma.

23

Symptoms

Uterine cancer is nearly painless in the initial stages. However, as the malignant tissue begins to grow, irregular bleeding and leukorrhea (usually after intercourse) appear. Leukorrhea gradually increases, becomes malodorous and laced with blood or pus, and causes itching in the vaginal area. Bleeding after intercourse should never be ignored. Advanced malignancy causes lower abdominal pain and, if the carcinoma has metastasized, pain in the affected areas. If the tumor spreads to the bladder or large intestine, the woman experiences incontinence or painful defecation; when it invades the peritoneum or pelvis, she feels pain in her legs. A woman with endometrial carcinoma suffers from recurrent pain, facial edema, and physical weakness, and looks extremely pale.

Treatment

At present, surgery is the only cure for uterine cancer. Because the uterus is an independent organ, it can be removed with no possibility of recurrence unless metastasis has already taken place. For this reason it is vitally important to detect early symptoms and begin treatment immediately. A gynecologist should diagnose and treat any abnormal hemorrhaging or leukorrhea. Steady bleeding indicates an advanced condition. Radiotherapy or chemotherapy can supplement surgery.

Chinese Herbal Formulas

Chinese herb formulas do not cure uterine cancer. The following formulas are supplemental therapy only and taken after surgery or if the patient refuses surgery.

*Cinnamon and Hoelen Formula with Coix
(*Kuei-chih-fu-ling-wan* with *I-yi-jen*) (6 Grams)
桂枝茯苓丸加薏苡仁

See page 15.

Uses
The primary stage of uterine cancer in the vigorous patient with a sensation of weight in the lower abdomen.

*_Tang-kuei_ and Gelatin Combination
(*Chiung-kuei-chiao-ai-tang*) 芎歸膠艾湯

See page 20.

Indications
Bleeding, anemia, a sensation of pressure in the lower abdomen, pain during intercourse.

*Ginseng and *Tang-kuei* Ten Combination
(*Shih-chuan-ta-pu-tang*) 十全大補湯

First recorded in the revised *Medical Dictionary of the Sung dynasty* (Tai ping huei min ho chi chu fang A.D. 1107-1110) by Chen Shih-wen and Pei Chung-yuan.

Herbal Components
3.0g ginseng	3.0g atractylodes	3.0g hoelen
3.0g cnidium	3.0g rehmannia	3.0g paeonia
3.0g cinnamon	3.0g *tang-kuei*	3.0g astragalus
1.0g licorice		

This formula consists of ten different herbs. Ginseng, atractylodes, hoelen, and licorice are strongly stomachic, nutritive herbs which improve the appetite and increase

25

digestive absorption. *Tang-kuei,* cnidium, paeonia, and rehmannia are hematinics which improve cardiac and liver
function, alleviate anemia and coarseness of the skin, and
improve circulation. Cinnamon and astragalus reinforce the
above actions.

Indications
Lack of vitality, anemia, weakness in various parts
of the body.

Uses
The patient who will not accept surgery but has severe
anemia, physical weakness, and malodorous leukorrhea.

*Ginseng and Longan Combination
(*Kuei-pi-tang*) 歸脾湯

See page 21.

Uses
Continuous bleeding, severe anemia, gastrointestinal
weakness, and stagnancy in the chest after taking Ginseng
and *Tang-kuei* Ten Combination.

4. Ovarian Tumors

Eighty percent of ovarian tumors are benign. The
tumors are called "sac tumors" because of their characteristic
sac shape. They vary in size from that of a fist to that of
an adult's head. The basic cause of ovarian tumors is unknown but they occur most frequently in women between
thirty and forty years of age.

Symptoms

Ovarian tumors are usually painless until they reach a certain size so they go unnoticed in the early stages. Occasional severe pain in the ovary occurs while the tumor is still small because of stagnant blood or bleeding of the tumor. If untreated, however, the tumor grows. By the time it reaches the size of a child's head it can be felt by palpation as a hard mass on the right or left side of the abdomen. At this stage, pressure on the rectum and bladder results in pain, constipation, and a sensation of heaviness in the lower abdomen. As it grows still larger, the benign tumor exerts pressure on the heart and lungs causing palpitations and labored breathing. General malnutrition is a concurrent symptom.

Treatment

Ovarian tumors should be surgically removed as soon after they are diagnosed as possible.

Chinese Herbal Formulas

*Persica and Rhubarb Combination
(*Tao-ho-cheng-chi-tang*) 桃核承氣湯

See page 16.

Uses
Severe symptoms due to a large tumor; constipation; pain in the abdomen.

27

*Cinnamon and Hoelen Formula (*Kuei-chih-fu-ling-wan*) 桂枝茯苓丸

See page 15.

Uses

Scanty menstrual flow.

5. Vaginal Trichomoniasis

Trichomonas vaginalis, a protozoan large enough to be seen with an ordinary microscope, is often present in small numbers in the normal, healthy vagina, but when present in large numbers, it causes vaginal trichomoniasis (trichomonal vaginitis). Once present it spreads easily by way of intercourse or by damp towels when bathing. Young girls, adult women, and elderly women are all vulnerable to this disease, and men may be asymptomatic carriers.

Symptoms

A copious, thin, yellow to yellowish-brown, very irritating, malodorous vaginal discharge; vulvovaginal burning and itching. In addition, the vaginal opening and wall turn fiery red. Bleeding may occur from the latter.

Treatment

Any questions about this disease should be referred to a gynecologist. The usual treatment is Flagyl metronidazole

taken orally under a doctor's supervision and with caution
because of possible side effects, especially in pregnant women
or those with liver disease. Douching removes the discharge
but cannot cure the infection. Women should abstain from
intercourse until completely cured to avoid infecting (or
reinfecting) their partner, or the man should use a condom.
If not completely cured, inflammation immediately reap-
pears. The infected woman's male partner should be checked
as a possible carrier of *Trichomonas* because the male urethra
and prostate are asymptomatic carrier sites.

Chinese Herbal Formulas

Licorice Root *(Glycyrrhizae radix)*
(Kan-tsao-i-wei) 甘草一味

First mentioned in the *Treatise on Febrile Diseases*
(Shang han lun).

Herbal Components
8.0 g licorice
This formula supplements energy, detoxifies, and loosens
phlegm when taken internally.

Uses
When the outside or external orifice of the vagina
has broken down, a dressing of licorice extract on the wound
checks the pain.

*Gentiana Combination
(Lung-tan-hsieh-kan-tang) 龍膽瀉肝湯

See page 14

Indications
Leukorrhea or external itching of the vagina.

6. Habitual Abortion

If a woman has three or more consecutive pregnancies ending in spontaneous abortions, usually at the same stage of pregnancy, she is said to suffer from habitual abortion, probably due to the same reason. Most abortions result from a hormone imbalance; a defective sperm or ovum; poor endometrial development (lining of the uterus); cervical weakness; congenital malformation or underdevelopment of the uterus; or incompatible blood types of husband and wife. Some 30% of habitual abortions are due to syphillis; other causes are diabetes, kidney disease, and tuberculosis. A medical examination can detect the cause and thus determine the appropriate precautions or treatment.

Symptoms

Spontaneous abortion most often occurs about three months after conception and is signalled by bleeding or cramps or both, lower back pain, and a heavy sensation in the legs. Abortion follows in a few days and, like childbirth, begins with grinding pain. If the abortion is complete, the bleeding stops after a few days. However, if the uterus is not completely emptied, the bleeding continues and there is danger of bacterial infection from the retained placenta The embryo is well-developed after five months and abortion at that point or later in the pregnancy is usually complete with no residual bleeding.

30

Treatment

Habitual abortion may often be prevented if the pregnant woman takes good care of herself. Helpful steps to avoid aborting are: (1) eat well and follow prenatal nutritional rules; (2) avoid hard physical work or excessive exercise; (3) stop or reduce smoking and consumption of alcohol; (4) try to maintain an even body temperature; (5) avoid prolonged constipation and diarrhea; (6) avoid exposure to influenza and infectious diseases; and (7) practice sexual moderation.

Chinese Herbal Formulas

Women having a weak and chill physique with an abnormally located uterus due to stagnant blood are prone to abort. Use of the proper Chinese formulas helps prevent habitual abortion. The following formulas are nutritives and tonics.

Tang-kuei and Paeonia Formula
(*Tang-kuei-shao-yao-san*) 當歸芍藥散

See page 18.

Indications
Cold limbs, headache, abdominal pain.

Uses
Weak conformations who continually abort.

*Tang-kuei and Evodia Combination
(*Wen-ching-tang*) 溫經湯

First recorded in the *Summaries of Household Remedies*
(Chin kuei yao lueh) by Chang Chung-ching (A.D. 142-
220).

Herbal Components
1.0g evodia	2.0g cinnamon	2.0g paeonia
3.0g *tang-kuei*	2.0g gelatin	2.0g licorice
2.0g cnidium	2.0g moutan	5.0g pinellia
2.0g ginseng	1.0g ginger	5.0g ophiopogon

Tang-kuei, paeonia, and cnidium are blood tonics. Gelatin
and ophiopogon nourish the blood. Ginseng and licorice
nourish *ch'i.* Evodia, ginger, and cinnamon relieve chills.
Pinellia stops leukorrhea and vomiting and, in conjunction
with ophiopogon, decreases flushing up. Moutan dispels
stagnant blood in the lower abdomen.

Indications
Weakness, fever, and thirst.

7. Toxemia of Pregnancy

Toxemia of pregnancy occurs in about 5% of pregnant
women, usually in women pregnant for the first time or
with preexisting hypertension or vascular disease. The cause
is unknown but is believed to be the failure of the mother s
body to adjust to the metabolic and physiological stresses
of pregnancy. Strenuous work and an improper diet are
also contributing factors. Toxemia in late pregnancy is
called pre-eclampsia.

Symptoms

Early symptoms are flushing or nausea in the mornings or an empty feeling in the stomach. The woman vomits food, gastric juice, and in severe cases, bile. She also has headaches, dizziness, occasional fever, and general tiredness. In pre-eclampsia, edema precedes the other symptoms, appearing first in the legs and then extending to the face and hands. In severe toxemia (eclampsia) the pregnant woman suffers from hypertension, albuminuria, oliguria, mental confusion, convulsions, and coma. Eclampsia is fatal if untreated.

Treatment

Prevention is the best treatment for toxemia. A pregnant woman should have regular examinations during the first five months of pregnancy; monthly examinations during the sixth, seventh, and eighth months; and weekly examinations during the ninth month. She should avoid mental or physical overexertion; eat sufficient amounts of complete, low-calorie protein such as eggs, meat, cheese, and bean curd, and other foods necessary to a well-balanced prenatal diet; eat enough small meals not to feel hungry; and avoid constipation. Because any disorder of pregnancy worsens with constipation, the woman should have a bowel movement every morning and eat generous amounts of vegetables. If constipation occurs, however, the use of enemas and cathartics should be avoided as they may induce abortion. A woman in the late stage of toxemia must have physical and mental quiet, ample rest, and normal salt intake, and must increase her consumption of water.

Chinese Herbal Formulas

* Minor Pinellia and Hoelen Combination
(*Hsiao-pan-hsia-chia-fu-ling-tang*) 小半夏加茯苓湯

First recorded in the *Summaries of Household Remedies* (Chin kuei yao lueh) of the Han dynasty.

Herbal Components
    8.0g pinellia   5.0g hoelen   1.0g ginger
Pinellia is an expectorant and antiemetic. Ginger is a stomachic. Hoelen and pinellia eliminate ascites and increase the flow of urine.

Uses
    "Morning sickness" -- vomiting and stomach discomfort.

*Hoelen Five Herb Formula
(*Wu-ling-san*) 五苓散

First mentioned in the medical dictionary of the Han dynasty, *Treatise on Febrile Diseases* (Shang han lun), *and Summaries of Household Remedies* (Chin kuei yao lueh A.D. 205).

Herbal Components
    6.5g hoelen   4.5g polyporus   4.5g atractylodes
    6.0g alisma   3.0g cinnamon
Alisma, polyporus, hoelen, and atractylodes relieve fluid accumulation in the stomach, increase the flow of urine, and dispel edema. Alisma and polyporus cure thirst. Cinnamon dispels surface heat, cures flushing up, and acts in conjunction with the other herbs as a diuretic.

Indications
    Dry throat, oliguria, edema, hypertension, severe albuminuria, headache, nausea.

*Bupleurum and Hoelen Combination
(*Chai-ling-tang*) 柴苓湯

First recorded in *Efficacious Prescriptions of Our Ancestors* (Shih i te hsiao fang) by Wei I-lin during the Yuan dynasty (A.D. 1260-1368).

Herbal Components
5.0g bupleurum	2.5g jujube	2.5g polyporus
4.0g pinellia	4.0g ginger	2.5g atractylodes
2.5g scute	2.0g licorice	2.5g hoelen
2.5g ginseng	2.5g cinnamon	4.0g alisma

Bupleurum relieves chest distention. Bupleurum and scute are antiphlogistics that dispel chest distention. Pinellia and ginger serve as antiemetics and appetizers. Ginseng, licorice, and jujube improve gastric function and relieve chest distention. Alisma, polyporus, hoelen, and atractylodes dispel "stagnant water" in the stomach and intestines, increase the flow of urine, and eliminate edema. Cinnamon dispels superficial fever, alleviates flushing up, and coordinates the diuretic actions of the other herbs.

Uses
    Conformation similar to that of Hoelen Five Herb Formula (*Wu-ling-san*) but with distention at the chest and heart, mild fever, headache, and nausea with anorexia.

*Capillaris Combination
(*Yin-chen-hao-tang*) 茵陳蒿湯

First recorded in the Chinese medical works *Treatise on Febrile Diseases* (Shang han lun) and *Summaries of House-*

35

hold Remedies (Chin kuei yao lueh) by Chang Chung-ching (A.D. 142-220).

Herbal Components
4.0g capillaris   3.0g gardenia   1.0g rhubarb
Capillaris is an antiphlogistic and diuretic, effective for stagnant heat and jaundice. Gardenia is also an antiphlogistic and diuretic, effective for stagnant heat, jaundice, and distention in the chest near the heart. Rhubarb is a laxative and antipyretic.

Indications
Fullness at the upper abdomen, distention at the chest and heart, thirst, constipation, dysuria, edema.

Uses
Sometimes, in combination with Hoelen Five Herb Formula (*Wu-ling-san*), better results are produced.

*Stephania and Ginseng Combination
(*Mu-fang-chi-tang*) 木防己湯

First written about in *Summaries of Household Remedies* (Chin kuei yao lueh) of the Han dynasty.

Herbal Components
4.0g stephania   3.0g ginseng
3.0g cinnamon   10.0g gypsum
Stephania increases blood circulation and dispels stagnant water in the chest. Gypsum and ginseng remove stress, thirst, and distention beneath the heart. Gypsum dispels stagnant water in the chest. Cinnamon removes flushing up and increases the flow of urine.

Indications
Distention at the heart, facial darkness, abdominal

fullness, gasping, palpitations, difficult breathing, distention
at the chest, edema, oliguria, thirst, a sunken pulse.

*Rehmannia Eight Formula
(*Pa-wei-ti-huang-wan*) 八味地黄丸

First mentioned in *Summaries of Household Remedies*
(Chin kuei yao lueh A.D. 205).

Herbal Components
8.0g rehmannia	4.0g dioscorea	4.0g cornus
3.0g hoelen	3.0g moutan	3.0g alisma
1.0g cinnamon	1.0g aconite	

The herbs in this formula have astringent, hematinic, and
nutritive properties. Rehmannia invigorates and nourishes.
Cornus is warming, invigorating, and strengthens the kidneys.

Uses
Edema with marked hypertension and albuminuria,
thirst, dysuria, flushing, and pain at the waist and feet.

*Hoelen and Alisma Combination
(*Fen-hsiao-tang*) 分消湯

First recorded in *Recovery from Myriad Diseases* (Wan
ping hui chun) of the Ming dynasty.

Herbal Components
5.0g atractylodes	2.0g polyporus	1.0g inula
2.5g hoelen	2.0g alisma	1.0g ginger
2.0g citrus	1.0g areca	1.0g juncus
1.0g cardamon	1.0g *chih-shih*	2.0g cyperus
2.0g magnolia bark		

A combination of Magnolia and Ginger Formula (*Pin-wei-*

san) and Hoelen and Polyporus Combination (*Szu-ling-tang*) and other herbs. Magnolia and Ginger Formula is good for problems of the stomach and spleen and for dispelling stagnant food and relieving ascites. *Szu-ling-tang* dispels moist heat in the stomach and treats dysuria (painful urination). *Chih-shih*, cyperus, areca, cardamon, and inula are aromatic stomachics and good for dispelling stagnant *ch'i*. Juncus is a diuretic and antipyretic that increases vitality and nourishes the spleen.

Uses

Mild edema of the limbs or face with obvious water stagnancy at the abdomen; hardened swelling at the abdomen (especially after a meal); a sunken, tense pulse.

Tang-kuei and Paeonia Formula
(*Tang-kuei-shao-yao-san*) 當歸芍藥散

See page 18.

Uses

A preventative and treatment for toxemia of pregnancy.

8. Postoperative Symptoms

Certain symptoms frequently occur after gynecological surgeries, such as a hysterectomy due to uterine myoma, the removal of an ovary (ovariotomy) because of a sac tumor or abnormal pregnancy, or a mastectomy due to breast cancer. Most of the women affected are slender and have cold hands and feet.

Symptoms

The woman will experience facial fever or fever of the torso, chills, dizziness, headaches, palpitations, and shoulder pain. After abdominal surgery, she will have abdominal pain, constipation, and a sensation of abdominal distention.

Chinese Herbal Formulas

*Cinnamon and Paeonia Combination
(*Kuei-chih-chia-shao-yao-tang*) 桂枝加芍藥湯

Recorded in the *Treatise on Febrile Diseases* (Shang han lun) of the Han dynasty.

Herbal Components

4.0g cinnamon	4.0g jujube	2.0g licorice
6.0g paeonia	4.0g ginger	

Cinnamon and ginger are stimulants; they improve blood circulation and functioning of the internal organs. Paeonia is a sedative and eases pain. Jujube and licorice are tonics.

Indications

Tense abdominal muscles and abdominal pain.

Tang-kuei, Evodia, and Ginger Combination
(*Tang-kuei-szu-ni-chia-wu-chu-yu-sheng-chiang-tang*)
當歸四逆加吳茱萸生薑湯

First recorded in the *Treatise on Febrile Diseases* (Shang han lun) by Chang Chung-ching of the Han dynasty.

Herbal Components

3.0g *tang-kuei*	2.0g asarum	5.0g jujube
3.0g cinnamon	2.0g licorice	2.0g evodia
3.0g paeonia	3.0g akebia	4.0g ginger

Tang-kuei and paeonia nourish the blood and increase blood circulation. Cinnamon and asarum remove internal chills. Akebia increases blood circulation. Jujube and licorice nourish *ch'i*. Evodia remedies flushing up, increases blood circulation, halts vomiting and headaches. Ginger, an acrid stomachic, relieves vomiting.

Indications

Abdominal distention, abdominal pain, chilling, and a tendency towards tiredness.

9. Mastitis

Mastitis is the inflammation of the breast. Acute suppurative mastitis in a nursing mother results from a staphylococcal infection, usually carried by the infant from the nursery. Infection is introduced through a nipple damaged by nursing. Stagnant mastitis results from milk stagnation or a mild deficiency in a nursing mother. Both of these types of mastitis can be brought on by an endocrine or autonomic nerve disorder. A nervous disorder sometimes causes an inflammative constitution and predisposes a woman towards bacterial infection.

Chronic cystic mastitis, a benign condition, is the most common disease affecting the breast. About 20% of all women develop breast cysts before menopause; new cysts seldom appear after menopause. Women with chronic cystic mastitis are nearly three times likelier to develop breast cancer later in life than women without cysts. The palpable masses in both breasts of these women should be examined around the time of menopause and frequently thereafter.

Important points to consider in treatment are the number of pregnancies the woman has had; the number, if any, of abortions; problems with breast feeding; and incidents of hormone injections in the past.

Symptoms

In suppurative mastitis, a portion of the breast hardens, swells, and becomes red, feverish and very painful. Severe symptoms are pus, headaches, loss of appetite, and fatigue.

In stagnant mastitis, the breast swells and reddens and becomes painful as the mammary glands harden. There is no pus, but some women develop a slight fever (about 38°C).

Chronic cystic mastitis often shows no symptoms although the cysts may be tender, in which case the woman may feel pain or premenstrual breast discomfort. Discovery of the cysts is usually accidental or through self-examination of the breasts.

Treatment

Suppurative mastitis developing within the first four weeks after delivery is usually penicillin resistant. Nursing women with mild infections must disinfect their nipples before breast feeding. Women with severe infections must stop nursing temporarily to treat the infection and prevent constant reinfection.

Women with stagnant mastitis should breast feed at regular intervals and empty the breast of any milk remaining after nursing, either manually or with a breast pump.

Chronic cystic mastitis rarely requires treatment.

Sedatives, antiphlogistics, or cold therapy may alleviate symptoms of pain, swelling, and nervousness.

41

Chinese Herbal Formulas

*Pueraria Combination with Gypsum
(*Ko-ken-tang-chia-shih-kao*) 葛根湯加石膏

First mentioned in the *Treatise on Febrile Diseases* (Shang han lun) and *Summaries of Household Remedies* (Chin kuei yao lueh).
Pueraria Combination has been famous in China since ancient times for its curative powers. A physician is considered extremely well versed in Chinese medicine if he can make full use of this versatile formula.

Herbal Components
8.0g pueraria	3.0g peony	1.0g ginger
4.0g *ma-huang*	4.0g jujube	gypsum
3.0g cinnamon	2.0g licorice	

Pueraria regulates blood circulation and intestinal function along with bowel evacuation. *Ma-huang* and licorice cure coughs and relieve skin contractions. Peony strengthens gastrointestinal function. Licorice detoxifies the liver. Jujube nourishes. Ginger, one of the major botanicals in the Chinese materia medica, promotes blood circulation. Gypsum reduces fever.

Uses
The primary stage of a cold with chills, fever, swelling, and pain. To treat colds in nursing mothers.

*Minor Bupleurum Combination
(*Hsiao-chai-hu-tang*) 小柴胡湯

Recorded in the *Treatise on Febrile Diseases* (Shang han lun) and *Summaries of Household Remedies* (Chin kuei yao lueh A.D. 205) by Chang Chung-ching of the Han dynasty.

Herbal Components

7.0g bupleurum	4.0g ginger	2.0g licorice
3.0g scute	5.0g pinellia	3.0g ginseng
3.0g jujube		

Bupleurum and scute are anti-inflammative and detoxicative and dispel chest distention. Pinellia and ginger remove fluid accumulated in the stomach and treat nausea, vomiting, and loss of appetite. A combination of ginseng, jujube, and licorice is stomachic and relieves the sensation of fullness beneath the heart. Bupleurum also nourishes the liver.

Indications

No appetite.

Uses

The patient who has a fever after taking Pueraria Combination with gypsum.

*Bupleurum and Schizonepeta Formula with Forsythia　十味敗毒散加連翹
(*Shih-wei-pai-tu-san-chia-lien-chiao*)

The original prescription of Bupleurum and Schizonepeta Formula was first modified by a famous Japanese surgeon, Kakou Seichiu, based on his own experience. S. Asata later added forsythia, after which it became a well-known remedy for dermatological disorders.

Herbal Components

3.0g bupleurum	2.0g hoelen	3.0g cherry bark
1.0g ginger	3.0g platycodon	1.0g licorice
2.0g siler	3.0g cnidium	1.0g schizonepeta
2.0g *tu-huo*	3.0g forsythia	

This formula is a detoxicative and can reinforce liver function. Bupleurum and ginger promote diaphoresis. *Tu-huo*, siler, and hoelen treat arthritis and rheumatism. Platycodon and cnidium increase the flow of urine and stop suppuration. Schizonepeta and cherry bark are detoxicatives. Licorice synthesizes the actions of the other herbs.

Uses

The patient who has taken Bupleurum and Schizonepeta Formula but still has fever and pus.

*Platycodon and Jujube Combination (*Pai-nung-tang*) 排膿湯

First recorded in *Summaries of Household Remedies* (Chin kuei yao lueh) by Chang Chung-ching (A.D. 142-220).

Herbal Components
        3.0g licorice   6.0g jujube
        4.0g platycodon   3.0g ginger
Platycodon prevents suppuration and also dispels pus. Licorice and jujube relieve acute symptoms and, in combination with ginger, improve the actions of the other herbs.

Uses

To discharge pus.

*Cinnamon and Hoelen Formula (*Kuei-chih-fu-ling-wan*) 桂枝茯苓丸

See page 15.

Uses

Taken by obese women of middle age with stagnant blood in the lower abdomen. For constipation, rhubarb (0.5-2.0g) is added.

*Persica and Rhubarb Combination
(*Tao-ho-cheng-chi-tang*) 桃核承氣湯

See page 16.

Uses

Aggravated stagnant blood in the lower abdomen, ruddy face, flushing up, headache, and severe constipation.

Lithospermum and Oyster Shell Combination
(*Tzu-ken-mu-li-tang*) 紫根牡蠣湯

From *A New Study of Dermatomycosis and Pellagra* (Mai li hsin shu A.D. 1786) by Katakura Tsurutoshi of Japan.

Herbal Components

5.0g *tang-kuei*	2.0g cimicifuga	1.0g licorice
3.0g paeonia	4.0g oyster shell	1.5g lonicera
3.0g cnidium	2.0g astragalus	3.0g lithospermum
1.5g rhubarb		

Lithospermum relieves "blood heat" and treats resistant tinea and severe ulcers. Lonicera and cimicifuga dispel "heat poisoning" and treat ulcers. Astragalus nourishes the blood and muscles, and dispels pus. *Tang-kuei,* paeonia, and cnidium are hematinics. Rhubarb helps evacuation. Licorice coordinates the actions of the other herbs.

Uses

Prolonged mastitis when breast cancer is not suspected.

Tang-kuei Sixteen Herb Combination
(*Shih-liu-wei-liu-chi-ying*) 十六味流氣飲

From the "Carbuncle" category in *Recovery from Myriad Diseases* (Wan ping hui chun) of the Ming dynasty (1368-1644).

Herbal Components
3.0g *tang-kuei*	2.0g angelica	2.0g *chih-ko*
3.0g cnidium	2.0g astragalus	2.0g areca seed
3.0g paeonia	2.0g saussurea	2.0g perilla
3.0g cinnamon	2.0g lindera	2.0g siler
3.0g ginseng	2.0g licorice	2.0g magnolia bark
3.0g platycodon		

Ginseng, astragalus, and licorice supplement *ch'i*. *Tang-kuei*, paeonia, and cnidium nourish the blood. Saussurea, areca seed, *chih-ko*, magnolia bark, and perilla regulate the *ch'i*. Lindera and siler destroy stagnant *ch'i*. Cinnamon and angelica disperse stagnant blood. Platycodon disperses pus and heightens the effectiveness of the other herbs.

Uses

Swelling due to stagnant *ch'i* and undiagnosed tumors; swelling of shoulders, neck, or limbs; and emphysema. It is effective for fibrocystic disease, intraductal papillomas, and breast cancer.

10. Breast Cancer

Breast cancer attacks and kills more women than any other kind of cancer. Environment, heredity (a family history of breast cancer), and hormonal activity seem to affect the incidence of breast cancer. It is also statistically linked to women who do not have children before their thirties or have no children; to women who have had several spontaneous abortions; to women who begin menstruating at an older age than normal; and to women who reach menopause earlier than normal. Incidence of breast cancer is highest around menopause, then rises again after the age of sixty-five.

Symptoms

All women should be aware of the symptoms of breast cancer. The cancer usually begins in the ducts of the milk glands and appears as a hard, painless lump, most commonly located in the upper, outer quadrant of the breast. As the lump grows, the skin of the breast may dimple or flatten, or the nipple may sink, flatten, or tilt. Bloody discharge from the nipple is rare. Discovery of breast cancer is usually through breast self-examination, best conducted at the same time after each menstrual cycle or on the same date each month. Women in and past menopause should be especially alert to any abnormalities.

The procedure for breast self-examination follows.

1.   Observe the nude upper body before a well-lit mirror. Compare the shapes of the breasts and search for dimpling, swelling, and changes in contour.

2.   Repeat with arms raised.

3.   Repeat with hands pressed firmly on hips to flex the chest muscles.

4.   Lie down with a pillow or folded towel beneath the left shoulder. Raise the left arm, put the hand behind the neck, and press the left breast in a circular motion with the flat of the right hand, starting at the outside and moving inwards toward the nipple in a spiral. Finally, gently squeeze the nipple to check for discharge.

5.   Repeat for the right breast.

Treatment

Like any other cancer, early detection and treatment of breast cancer greatly improves the chances of a complete cure. Since 60-80% of biopsies of breast lumps are non-cancerous however, a woman need not be unduly worried when the doctor orders a biopsy. If biopsy shows the lump to be cancerous, the breast is usually removed. Where surgery is not feasible, radiation therapy may be used instead.

Chinese Herbal Formulas

*Cinnamon and Hoelen Formula
(*Kuei-chih-fu-ling-wan*) 桂枝茯苓丸

See page 15.

Uses

Edema of the legs, fever, constipation, and related symptoms.

Tang-kuei Sixteen Herb Combination
(*Shih-liu-wei-liu-chi-yin*) 十六味流氣飲

See page 46.

Uses

Edema of the legs, fever, constipation, and related symptoms.

11. Leukorrhea

Leukorrhea is a white or yellowish mucous discharge from the vagina or cervical canal. Since the vagina needs secretions to moisturize it, a certain amount of leukorrhea is normal, especially just before and just after menstruation, or during pregnancy. Constant leukorrhea, however, is often a sign of abnormality, usually infection of the lower reproductive tract. Leukorrhea in post-menopausal women may be a symptom of uterine cancer. Abnormal leukorrhea (changes in normal amount, color, consistency, or odor) may well indicate disease or signal a spontaneous abortion, expecially if mixed with pus or blood. Because the female genital tract is easily affected by disease or infection, it is important to neither ignore nor be ashamed of abnormal leukorrhea. A doctor's examination is needed to determine and treat the underlying cause.

Treatment

The underlying cause needs to be treated. Douching cleanses the vagina and may ease accompanying symptoms, such as itching, but should be done only on a doctor's advice because it can aggravate some conditions.

Chinese Herbal Formulas

*Gentiana Combination
(*Lung-tan-hsieh-kan-tang*) 龍膽瀉肝湯

See page 14.

49

Uses

Strong conformations with bladder inflammation, urethritis, and uteritis with severe heat; leukorrhea with a yellow or red color due to endometritis; vaginitis; or vaginal trichomoniasis.

Tang-kuei and Eight Herb Formula (*Pa-wei-tai-hsia-fang*) 八味帶下方

See page 17.

Uses

Chronic leukorrhea with a white or yellow color accompanied by moderate anemia and abdominal laxity; leukorrhea caused by gonococci or vaginal trichomoniasis.

*Cinnamon and Hoelen Formula (*Kuei-chih-fu-ling-wan*) 桂枝茯苓丸

See page 15.

Uses

Acute or chronic leukorrhea laced with blood, a feeling of pressure at the lower abdomen.

Tang-kuei and Paeonia Formula (*Tang-kuei-shao-yao-san*) 當歸芍藥散

See page 18.

Uses
     Weak conformations with leukorrhea of a white color
and a tendency towards anemia.

Lotus Seed Combination
(*Ching-hsin-lien-tzu-yin*) 清心蓮子飲

First mentioned in *The Medical Dictionary of the Sung
Dynasty* (Tai ping huei min ho chi chu fang A.D. 1107-
1110).

Herbal Components
     4.0g lotus seed   3.0g ginseng   2.0g astragalus
     4.0g ophiopogon 3.0g plantago   2.0g lycium bark
     4.0g hoelen   3.0g scute   2.0g licorice
The formula nourishes the spleen, stomach, and kidneys
and dispels "internal heat" in the heart and the lungs. Ophiopogon and lotus seed dispel "internal heat" in the heart and
nourish the heart and blood. Plantago and lycium bark
remove "internal heat" from the kidneys. Ginseng, astragalus,
lycium bark, scute, and ophiopogon remove "internal heat"
from the lungs and nourish the kidneys. Ginseng, hoelen,
and licorice nourish and invigorate the spleen and the
stomach.

Uses
     Chronic, very watery leukorrhea with gastrointestinal
weakness, physical chills, and weakness.

Tang-kuei and Magnolia Formula
(*Wu-chi-san*) 五積散

First recorded in *The Medical Dictionary of the Sung Dynasty* (Tai ping huei min ho chi chu fang A.D. 1107-1110).

Herbal Components

1.2g angelica	2.0g hoelen	1.2g *ma-huang*
2.0g citrus	1.2g platycodon	1.2g ginger
2.0g atractylodes	1.2g cinnamon	1.2g *tang-kuei*
1.2g *chih-ko*	1.2g licorice	1.2g magnolia bark
1.2g cnidium	2.0g pinellia	1.2g jujube
1.2g paeonia		

This formula combines three separate formulas. The atractylodes, citrus, licorice, and magnolia bark of Magnolia and Ginger Formula (*Ping-wei-san*) remove stagnant food. The pinellia, hoelen, citrus, licorice, and ginger of Citrus Combination with *chih-ko* (*Erh-chen-tang*) remove stagnant water in the stomach and watery sputum. The *tang-kuei*, paeonia, and cnidium of *Szu-wu-tang* nourish the blood and *ch'i*. Cinnamon, ginger, *ma-huang*, angelica, and platycodon are carminatives (expel gas) and increase blood circulation.

Uses

Diluted leukorrhea due to a cold; leukorrhea due to chilling from an air-conditioned room or exercising.

Bupleurum and Paeonia Formula (Chia-wei-hsiao-yao-san) 加味逍遙散

See page 19.

Uses

For those who have taken *Tang-kuei* and Peony Formula (*Tang-kuei-shao-yao-san*) in vain.

*Bupleurum and Dragon Bone Combination
(*Chai-hu-chia-lung-ku-mu-li-tang*) 柴胡加龍骨牡蠣湯

First mentioned in the *Treatise on Febrile Diseases* (Shang han lun A.D. 205) by Chang Chung-ching.

Herbal Components

5.0g bupleurum	2.5g ginger	2.5g jujube
4.0g pinellia	3.0g cinnamon	1.0g rhubarb
3.0g hoelen	2.5g ginseng	2.5g scute
2.5g oyster shell	2.5g dragon bone (*Draconis os*)	

The principal herbs of this formula are bupleurum, dragon bone, and hoelen. Bupleurum purges inner heat at the chest. Dragon bone soothes and sedates inner agitation. Hoelen is diuretic and calms the nerves. Bupleurum and scute relieve heat and stagnancy in the chest. Dragon bone and oyster shell sedate chest and abdominal palpitations, cardiac hyperfunction, insomnia, and fearfulness. Cinnamon cures flushing up. A combination of hoelen, pinellia, and ginger dispels fluid accumulated in the stomach. Rhubarb purges the intestines, draws out infection, and sedates. Jujube and ginger assist and reinforce the actions of the other herbs.

Uses

Leukorrhea.

*Ginseng and *Tang-kuei* Ten Combination
(*Shih-chuan-ta-pu-tang*) 十全大補湯

See page 25.

Uses

Physical weakness, lack of vigor, anemia, tendency towards fatigue, weak pulse, and continuous leukorrhea after childbirth or abortion.

53

*Ginseng and Ginger Combination
(*Jen-sheng-tang*) 人參湯

First mentioned in the *Treatise on Febrile Diseases* (Shang han lun) and *Summaries of Household Remedies* (Chin kuei yao lueh) by Chang Chung-ching.

Herbal Components

3.0g ginseng	3.0g ginger
3.0g licorice	3.0g atractylodes

The formula is called *Jen-sheng-tang* in *Summaries of Household Remedies* (Chin kuei yao lueh). In the *Treatise on Febrile Diseases* (Shang han lun) it is called *li* (to regulate) *chung* (the middle) *tang* (tea), or "to regulate the middle burning place" (spleen and stomach). Ginseng, the principal herb, nourishes and warms the spleen and stomach, strengthens gastrointestinal function, promotes metabolism, improves physical strength, and has sedative, diurectic, and antifatigue properties. Ginger assists ginseng in warming the spleen and stomach. Atractylodes relieves ascites. Licorice relieves pain. In short, the formula is excellent for weak digestion, malabsorption, and poor metabolism.

Uses

Leukorrhea with chilling. If the patient has gastrointestinal weakness, Major Six Herb Combination (*Liu-chun-tzu-tang*) may also be given.

Tang-kuei and Evodia Combination
(*Wen-ching-tang*) 溫經湯

See page 32.

Indications

Weakness, fever, and thirst.

Uses
For watery leukorrhea with chills at the waist.

12. Chills

Different kinds of chills affect mostly women younger than twenty years of age or women past menopause. Some women feel cold all over; others have cold feet or hands; others feel ice-cold in the back, stomach, and waist areas. Some feel cold around their heads while others feel cold at the backs of their knees but their faces feel hot. Some women often have cold hands, feet, and waist during the day, and feel cold at the waist for a long time after going to bed at night, even when the rest of their body is warm. The basic cause of such chills remains obscure. Blood circulation disturbed by a change in the nerve fibers or stagnant blood is one possible cause. Anemia might be another. A cold feeling limited to certain areas of the body might be caused by an imbalance in body fluids, a metabolic or autonomic nervous system disorder, gastrointestinal weakness, gastroptosis (downward displacement of the stomach), or even a general lack of vitality.

Chills are classified according to the area of the body affected and the severity of the sensation. Possible causes would then be assigned according to these factors.

1.   Chills at the waist and legs are caused by menopausal disorders, difficult menstruation, endometritis (inflammation of the endometrium), or uterine myoma (a tumor containing muscle tissue).

2.   Low temperature in one part of the body is caused by anemia, hypotension, heart disease, or an autonomic nervous system disorder.

3. A normal body temperature but a cold feeling is caused by nervousness, hysteria, or other emotional factors.

Treatment

If a specific problem or disease is causing the chills, it is treated first. Otherwise, sedatives may stabilize blood circulation and relax the nerves. Vitamin B is good for the nerves and vitamin E aids dilation of the blood vessels. The most important therapy, of course, is to keep the body warm.

Chinese Herbal Formula

*Tang-kuei and Paeonia Formula (*Tang-kuei-shao-yao-san*) 當歸芍藥散

See page 18.

Indications
Waist chills, leg chills, a sensation of tiredness, and a tendency towards anemia; also headache, dizziness, and shoulder ache.

Uses
Chills due to anemia.

Tang-kuei, Evodia, and Ginger Combination (*Tang-kuei-szu-ni-chia-wu-chu-yu-sheng-chiang-tang*) 當歸四逆加吳茱萸生薑湯

See page 39.

Uses
      Chills in women past middle age, especially chilling of
the hands and feet; stagnant blood in the limbs with
chilblain; a weak and sunken pulse; abdominal fullness;
abdominal pain and hernia.

*Hoelen and Ginger Combination
(*Ling-chiang-chu-kan-tang*) 苓薑朮甘湯

First recorded in *Summaries of Household Remedies* (Chin
kuei yao lueh) by Chang Chung-ching (A.D. 142-220).

Herbal Components
      6.0g hoelen   3.0g atractylodes
      3.0g ginger   2.0g licorice
Ginger is warm in nature and acts as a diuretic. Hoelen and
atractylodes increase *ch'i* and dispel superficial water. Licorice and ginger are tonics and treat frequent urination.

Uses
      Severe chilling from waist to feet; polyuria in those
having normal upper body temperature.

Vitality Combination
(*Chen-wu-tang*) 眞武湯

First recorded in *Treatise on Febrile Diseases* (Shang han lun)
by Chang Chung-ching (A.D. 142-220).

Herbal Components
      5.0g hoelen   3.0g atractylodes   1.0g aconite
      3.0g paeonia   3.0g ginger
Hoelen and atractylodes dispel ascites and promote gastroin-

testinal function. Paeonia relieves muscle tension, spasms, and pain. Aconite and ginger improve metabolism and increase vitality.

Uses

Metabolic disorders, lack of vigor, tendency towards fatigue, chilling at the hands and feet, water stagnancy at the abdomen, and pain and diarrhea from the cold. Note: When chilling is associated with neuralgia and rheumatism, the patient should take Aconite Combination (*Fu-tzu-tang*).

Aconite, Ginseng, and Ginger Combination
(*Fu-tzu-li-chung-tang*) 附子理中湯

First recorded in *Treatise on Febrile Diseases* (Shang han lun) by Chang Chung-ching (A.D. 142-220).

Herbal Components
3.0g ginseng   3.0g licorice   3.0g ginger
3.0g atractylodes   0.5-1.0g aconite

Ginseng, ginger, licorice, and atractylodes nourish *ch'i* and the spleen, and dispel chills. Aconite warms the body and improves metabolic functioning.

Uses

Gastrointestinal weakness, gastroptosis, emaciation, lack of vigor, mild anemia, and general chilling. For severe chills, Ginseng, Ginger, and Aconite Combination (*Fu-tzu-li-chung-tang*) is recommended.

Aconite and G.L. Combination
(*Szu-ni-tang*) 四逆湯

First recorded in *Treatise on Febrile Diseases* (Shang han

lun) and *Summaries of Household Remedies* (Chin kuei yao lueh) by Chang Chung-ching (A.D. 142-220).

Herbal Components
    3.0g licorice   2.0g ginger   0.5-1.0g aconite
Aconite is a stimulant that increases vitality. Ginger dispels chills. Licorice is an analgesic, expectorant, and antidysenteric.

Uses
    Severe chilling of the hands and feet; following diarrhea when the patient has severe chills, weak and sunken pulse, pale face, and fatigue.

13. Blood Stagnation

    Blood stagnation is characterized by mental and emotional disorders brought on by menstruation, pregnancy, childbirth, puerperal fever, abortion, menopause, or some methods of contraception. Common autonomic nervous system symptoms are a ruddy face, congestion, sweating followed by chills, fever in the arms and legs, a sensation of pressure at the heart, palpitations, fluctuating blood pressure, vertigo, and tinnitus (a ringing sound in the ears). Emotional symptoms are nervousness, excitability, hysteria, melancholy, confusion, amnesia, headaches, shoulder stiffness, and a tendency to tire easily. Young women commonly exhibit a sensation of chills. Blood stagnation in middle-aged women is usually from menopausal disorders.
    Because blood stagnation is an emotional disorder, the removal or reduction of sources of stress may markedly reduce the symptoms. Tranquilizers are sometimes useful

59

and Chinese herb formulas are prescribed according to blood, *ch'i*, or water stagnation. (See Introduction for full explanation of this important concept of Chinese medicine.)

Chinese Herbal Formulas

Cinnamon and Hoelen Formula (Kuei-chih-fu-ling-wan) 桂枝茯苓丸

See page 15.

Uses

Resistance and pain when pressed on the lower abdomen around the umbilicus--the symptoms of stagnant blood, pelvic congestion, headache, abdominal pain, and menstrual difficulties in a strong conformation. Most patients are vigorous with a ruddy face. Those having constipation should add rhubarb (1.5-2.0g) to this formula. In severe cases, Persica and Rhubarb Combination (*Tao-ho-cheng-chi-tang*) is recommended.

Tang-kuei and Paeonia Formula (*Tang-kuei-shao-yao-san*) 當歸芍藥散

See page 18.

Uses

Weak women with a tendency towards anemia and fatigue, chilling at the waist and feet, heaviness of the head, vertigo, tinnitus, palpitations, and aching in the lower abdomen.

60

*Bupleurum and Paeonia Formula
(*Chia-wei-hsiao-yao-san*) 加味逍遙散

See page 19.

Uses

Chills in chronic and weak conformations.

Tang-kuei Four Combination
(*Szu-wu-tang*) 四物湯

The all-purpose herb tea for gynecological diseases, it has been mainly used by women but is sometimes given to men as well. First recorded in the *Medical Dictionary of the Sung Dynasty* (Tai ping huei min ho chi chu fang A.D. 1107-1110).

Herbal Components

4.0g *tang-kuei*   4.0g cnidium   4.0g paeonia
4.0g rehmannia

Rehmannia is hematinic. *Tang-kuei* regulates vitality and supplements the blood; cnidium improves blood circulation and vitality. Paeonia harmonizes the blood.

Uses

Anemia and nervousness and gynecological diseases. Not for people with diarrhea.

*Bupleurum and Dragon Bone Combination
(*Chai-hu-chia-lung-ku-mu-li-tang*) 柴胡加龍骨牡蠣湯

See page 53.

Uses

A sedative for pressure at the chest, uncomfortable feeling at the umbilicus, palpitations, congestion, headache, vertigo, insomnia, and fatigue due to blood diseases.

Bupleurum, Citrus, and Pinellia Formula
(*I-kan-san-chia-chen-pi-pan-hsia*) 抑肝散加陳皮半夏

Herbal Components

3.0g *tang-kuei*	4.0g atractylodes	1.5g licorice
3.0g gambir	4.0g hoelen	3.0g citrus
3.0g cnidium	2.0g bupleurum	5.0g pinellia

Gambir is an anti-spasmodic effective in relieving spasms of the limbs. *Tang-kuei* nourishes hepatic blood. Cnidium improves blood circulation. Bupleurum with licorice and gambir sedates and alleviates excessive liver *ch'i*. Hoelen and atractylodes are diuretics which release stagnant water from the stomach. Citrus and pinellia are expectorants.

Uses

Nervousness with epilepsy; anxiety accompanied by proneness to anger; and insomnia.

*Cinnamon and Dragon Bone Combination
(*Kuei-chih-chia-lung-ku-mu-li-tang*)
桂枝加龍骨牡蠣湯

Recorded in *Summaries of Household Remedies* (Chin kuei yao lueh) of the Han dynasty.

Herbal Components

4.0g cinnamon	4.0g ginger	3.0g oyster shell
4.0g paeonia	2.0g licorice	4.0g jujube
3.0g dragon bone		

Kuei-chih-tang relieves muscular tension and nourishes yin and yang. Cinnamon is a nutrient. Paeonia nourishes yin. Ginger relieves chills. Licorice and jujube nourish the spleen and *ch'i* Dragon bone constricts yang. Oyster shell constricts yin.

Uses
    Nervousness, congestion, headache, insomnia, palpitation, fearfulness, sweating, night sweats, and a tendency towards physical weakness.

*Licorice and Jujube Combination
(Kan-mai-ta-tsao-tang)* 甘麥大棗湯

First mentioned in *Summaries of Household Remedies* (Chin kuei yao lueh) by Chang Chung-ching (A.D. 142-220) of the Han dynasty.

Herbal Components
    3.0g licorice   2.5g jujube   14.0g wheat
Licorice and jujube treat muscle spasms, nervous excitability, and various pains. Wheat relieves excitability.

Indications
    Hysteria, nervousness, spasms, insomnia, tendency towards yawning, and in severe cases coma or mania.

Coptis and Scute Combination
(Huang-lien-chieh-tu-tang) 黃連解毒湯

First recorded in *A Pocket Book of Emergency Prescriptions* (Chou hou pei chi fang) by Ko Hung during the Chin dynasty (A.D. 281-341).

Herbal Components

3.0g scute	1.5g phellodendron
1.5g coptis	2.0g gardenia

Coptis dispels "internal heat" in the heart, spleen, and stomach, and relieves distention beneath the heart and palpitations. Scute dispels "internal heat" in the lungs and intestines and reduces inflammation, congestion, hemoptysis, and bleeding. Phellodendron is a diuretic and astringent effective for "internal heat" in the kidneys and bladder. Gardenia is a sedative, hemostatic, and antiemetic.

Uses

Ruddy face, congestion, insomnia, stress, palpitations, and stagnant blood.

Vitality Combination
(Chen-wu-tang) 眞武湯

See page 57.

Uses

A weak conformation with proneness to becoming tired, chilling, weak pulse and abdomen, stagnancy in the gastrointestinal tract, decrease in urinary output, abdominal pain and diarrhea, and vertigo or palpitations.

14. Menstrual Problems

The average menstrual cycle is approximately thirty days. Frequent menstruation (a short cycle, less than twenty-one days) and scarce menstruation (a long cycle, more than forty days) are considered menstrual aberrations. However, if a women's menstrual cycle is regular and she is healthy, then the length, whether short or long, is normal for her. Most irregularities appear during adolescence, lactation, or menopause.

Frequent menstruation (polymenorrhea) can be caused by uterine inflammation, swelling, or retroflexion, or by abnormal ovarian function. Women with such cycles often have extended periods of heavy bleeding (from one week to ten days) which can result in anemia and weakness. Some women become more or less hysterical.

Other menstrual problems include amenorrhea (absence of menstruation), dysmenorrhea (painful menstruation), and scarce, scanty, excessive, precocious (onset before the age of nine), and vicarious menstruation.

The causes of amenorrhea range from genetic factors and hormonal, nutritional, or psychological factors to disease. Since the possible causes of abnormal menstrual cycles vary widely, they often can be determined only by extensive testing.

Vicarious menstruation is cyclic bleeding from the nose, mouth, bladder, stomach, conjuctiva, or skin due to the cyclic rise and fall in serum estrogen levels. Vicarious nasal menstruation alone accounts for 30% of nonuterine cyclic bleeding and is caused by cyclic vascular congestion and hyperemia of the nasal mucous membranes. (Hyperemia is increased blood in a part of the body resulting in distention of the blood vessels.)

Painful menstruation (or cramps) severe enough to interfere with a woman's everyday life is called dysmenorrhea. Dysmenorrhea caused by an inflammation, such as endometritis, is alleviated by curing the infection. The basic causes of essential dysmenorrhea include:

1   Ovulation and excessive production of prostaglandins which in some women cause uterine hyperactivity. Uterine tension, strong contractions, and a decreased blood flow to the uterus cause the greatest pain.

2.   A constitutional predisposition to over-respond to potentially painful stimuli (a low pain threshold).
    ~ 3.   Psychological factors such as general anxiety or tension.

Treatment

Psychiatric counseling is necessary only when the cause is psychological. Otherwise, simple analgesics or pro-staglandin synthetase inhibitors, such as ibuprofen (used under a doctor's supervision because of possible side effects), usually control pain. Antiemetics or mild tranquilizers are helpful in some cases, and oral contraceptives have been used to produce anovulatory cycles. A complete understanding of the process that causes the cramps and an attempt to continue normal activities help many women endure the pain when it cannot be avoided.

The most common treatment for menstrual problems is hormone therapy by a qualified physician. A calm, controlled attitude on the part of the doctor and patient may ease resulting mental distress.

Chinese Herbal Formulas

*Tang-kuei and Paeonia Formula (Tang-kuei-shao-yao-san) 當歸芍藥散

See page 18.

Uses
    Difficult menstruation due to an ill-developed uterus or narrow cervical opening; anemia and chilling.

*Cinnamon and Hoelen Formula
(*Kuei-chih-fu-ling-wan*) 桂枝茯苓丸

See page 15.

Uses

Anteflexion or retroflexion of the uterus, uterine myoma, resistant pain when pressed on the lower abdomen, and pelvic congestion.

*Persica and Rhubarb Combination
(*Tao-ho-cheng-chi-tang*) 桃核承氣湯

See page 16.

Uses

Difficult menstruation due to inflammation, post-menstrual pain, and hemorrhage; cramping and pain when pressed on the lower abdomen, and congestion. In severe cases, purge after taking this formula for two or three days, and then take Cinnamon and Persica Combination (*Che-chung-yin*). The condition will be improved by using this therapy for several months.

*Minor Cinnamon and Paeonia Combination
(*Hsiao-chien-chung-tang*) 小建中湯

First mentioned in the medical works of the Han dynasty, *Treatise on Febrile Diseases* (Shang han lung) and *Summaries of Household Remedies* (Chin kuei yao lueh) by Chang Chung-ching (A.D. 142-220).

67

Herbal Components

6.0g paeonia	4.0g licorice	20.0g maltose
4.0g cinnamon	4.0g jujube	2.0g ginger

Maltose and jujube have nutritive effects. Licorice relieves prominent symptoms; in combination with paeonia, its analgesic effects are improved. Cinnamon with licorice stops palpitations. Ginger is a stomachic and promotes absorption of the herbs.

Uses

A lack of vitality, anemia, physical weakness, and difficult menstruation due to an ill-developed uterus. The patient who has a tendency towards fatigue, chilling, and spasms around abdominal muscles should add *tang-kuei* (4.0g).

Cinnamon and Hoelen Formula (Kuei-chih-fu-ling-wan) 桂枝茯苓丸

See page 15.

Uses

Scarce menstruation.

Tang-kuei and Paeonia Formula (*Tang-kuei-shao-yao-san*) 當歸芍藥散

See page 18.

Uses

Both frequent and scarce menstruation.

Tang-kuei Four Combination
(*Szu-wu-tang*) 四物湯

See page 61.

Uses

Amenorrhea before menopause in women with defective uterine development, malfunctioning ovaries, or an atrophied endometrium.

*Bupleurum and Paeonia Formula
(*Chia-wei-hsiao-yao-san*) 加味逍遙散

See page 19.

Uses

Menopausal symptoms, physical weakness, or a long-standing tendency towards anemia or tuberculosis; developmental uterine defects. Addition of 3.0g each of rehmannia and cyperus enhance the formula.

*Ginseng and *Tang-kuei* Ten Combination
(*Shih-chuan-ta-pu-tang*) 十全大補湯

See page 25.

Uses

Amenorrhea and anemia caused by generalized fatigue, prolonged lactation, or massive hemorrhage during childbirth. If there is anorexia after taking this formula, the patient should take Ginseng and Longan Combination (*Kuei-pi-tang*) or Ginseng and Astragalus Combination (*Pu-chung-i-chi-tang*)

*Cinnamon and Hoelen Formula
(*Kuei-chih-fu-ling-wan*) 桂枝茯苓丸

See page 15.

*Persica and Rhubarb Combination
(*Tao-ho-cheng-chi-tang*) 桃核承氣湯

See page 16.

Uses

Uteritis or endometritis; resistant pain when pressed on the lower abdomen--stagnant blood; excessive and vicarious menstruation. For constipation, add rhubarb (0.5 - 2.0g). In severe cases with congestion, headache, and ruddy face, the patient should take Persica and Rhubarb Combination.

*Rhubarb and Moutan Combination
(*Ta-huang-mu-tan-pi-tang*) 大黃牡丹皮湯

See page 17.

Uses

Stagnant blood and distention of the abdomen due to amenorrhea.

*Bupleurum and Cinnamon Combination
(*Chai-hu-kuei-chih-tang*) 柴胡桂枝湯

First mentioned in the medical works of the Han dynasty,

Treatise on Febrile Diseases (Shang han lun) and *Summaries of Household Remedies* (Chin kuei yao lueh) by Chang Chung-ching (A.D. 142-220).

Herbal Components

5.0g bupleurum	4.0g pinellia	1.5g licorice
2.5g cinnamon	2.0g scute	2.0g ginseng
2.5g paeonia	2.0g jujube	1.0g ginger

This combination consists of a combination of Minor Bupleurum Combination (*Hsiao-chai-hu-tang*) and Cinnamon Combination (*Kuei-chih-tang*). Bupleurum promotes blood circulation in the liver and relieves chest distention and moist heat. Scute dispels heat in the chest and may be given for inflammation of the digestive organs. Ginseng improves the functioning of internal organs and increases appetite. Ginger and pinellia arrest vomiting, decrease expectoration, increase appetite and flow of urine, and dispel edema in the stomach and chest. Cinnamon cures "flushing" and headache. Paeonia stimulates the action of the digestive organs and acts as a nutrient when in combination with jujube, ginger, and licorice.

Uses

Distention at the chest and amenorrhea due to tension in the lower abdomen. Rhubarb (0.5-2.0g) added to this formula relieves chest distention and helps restore menstruation. For severe cases in strong women, Major Bupleurum Combination (*Ta-chai-hu-tang*) is recommended.

Tang-kuei and Gelatin Combination (*Chiung-kuei-chiao-ai-tang*) 芎歸膠艾湯

See page 20.

71

Uses

Vicarious menstruation, tendency towards anemia, and physical weakness due to chills; excessive menstruation.

*Stephania and Astragalus Combination
(*Fang-chi-huang-chi-tang*) 防己黃耆湯

First mentioned in *Summaries on Household Remedies* (Chin kuei yao lueh) by Chang Chung-ching (A.D. 142-220).

Herbal Components
5.0g·stephania   3.0g jujube   3.0g atractylodes
5.0g astragalus   1.5g licorice   3.0g ginger

Stephania and atractylodes cure edema, stop excessive perspiration, increase the flow of urine, and relieve pain. Astragalus and licorice nourish the skin. Jujube and licorice improve the taste and coordinate the actions of the other herbs. Ginger acts as a stomachic (a substance which stimulates the digestive activity of the stomach).

Uses

Obese women with a tendency to tire easily and scanty menstruation (every two or three months).

15. Menopausal Disorders

In menopause a woman's ovaries gradually cease to function and hence she loses the ability to bear children.

The onset of menopause is sometimes abrupt but more often gradual, usually occurring between the ages of forty and fifty. This winding down period usually lasts from one to three years and during this time ovulation and menstruation become irregular and finally stop altogether. As ovarian function fluctuates, an estrogen deficiency disrupts hypothalamic control of the autonomic nervous system and one out of five women experience hot flashes. Psychological and physiological reactions cause symptoms such as chills, nervousness, palpitations, insomnia, depression, irritability, headaches or other somatic aches, or a change in appetite. Some women also have painful menstruation and almost all women have some menstrual irregularities.

Treatment

Menopausal disorders are not pathological. Tranquilizers, sedatives, or hormone replacement therapy may be prescribed, but most women need minimal medical and emotional therapy during this natural process.

Chinese Herbal Formulas

*Cinnamon and Hoelen Formula
(*Kuei-chih-fu-ling-wan*) 桂枝茯苓丸

See page 15.

Uses
Resistance and pain when pressed on the lower abdomen around the umbilicus—symptoms of stagnant blood—pelvic congestion, headache, abdominal pain, and menstrual difficulties in a strong conformation. Most of the patients are vigorous and have a ruddy face. Those having

73

constipation should add rhubarb (0.5-2.0g). For severe cases, Persica and Rhubarb Combination is prescribed.

*Tang-kuei and Paeonia Formula
(*Tang-kuei-shao-yao-san*) 當歸芍藥散

See page 18.

Uses
Weak women with a tendency towards anemia and fatigue, chilling at the waist and feet, heaviness of head, vertigo, tinnitus, palpitations, and aching in the lower abdomen.

*Bupleurum and Paeonia Formula
(*Chia-wei-hsiao-yao-san*) 加味逍遙散

See page 19.

Uses
Semi-strong and semi-weak conformation: obvious complications of blood disease, such as fever and chilling; fever in the limbs; heaviness of head; vertigo; ruddy face; night sweats; insomnia; generalized tiredness; and loss of appetite.

Tang-kuei Four Combination
(*Szu-wu-tang*) 四物湯

See page 61.

Uses
An excellent formula for gynecological diseases, anemia, and nervousness. A patient with diarrhea should not take it.

*Bupleurum and Dragon Bone Combination
(Chai-hu-chia-lung-ku-mu-li-tang) 柴胡加龍骨牡蠣湯

See page 53.

Uses
A sedative to be taken for pressure at the chest, uncomfortable feeling at the umbilicus, palpitations, flushing up, headache, vertigo, insomnia, and fatigue due to blood diseases.

*Bupleurum, Citrus, and Pinellia Formula
(I-kan-san-chia-chen-pi-pan-hsia) 抑肝散加陳皮半夏

See page 62.

Uses
Nervousness with epilepsy; anxiety accompanied by proneness to anger; and insomnia.

*Pinellia and Magnolia Combination
(Pan-hsia-hou-pu-tang) 半夏厚朴湯

See page 91.

Uses
Weak patients with a sensation of something blocking or itching and stimulating the throat, a hoarse voice, a

75

weak and sunken pulse, and a patting sound at the lower part of the heart.

*Cinnamon and Dragon Bone Combination (*Kuei-chih-chia-lung-ku-mu-li-tang*)

桂枝加龍骨牡蠣湯

See page 62.

Uses

Nervousness, congestion, headache, insomnia, palpitations, fearfulness, sweating, night sweats, and a tendency towards physical weakness.

*Licorice and Jujube Combination (*Kan-mai-ta-tsao-tang*) 甘麥大棗湯

See page 71.

Uses

Hysteria, nervousness, spasms, insomnia, tendency to yawn, and in severe cases coma or mania.

Coptis and Scute Combination (*Huang-lien-chieh-tu-tang*) 黃連解毒湯

See page 63.

Uses

A ruddy face, congestion, insomnia, stress, palpitations, and blood stagnation.

Vitality Combination
(*Chen-wu-tang*) 眞武湯

See page 57.

Uses

A weak conformation with proneness to becoming tired, chilling, weak pulse and abdomen, stagnancy in the gastrointestinal tract, decrease in urinary output, abdominal pain and diarrhea, and vertigo or palpitations.

Tang-kuei, Evodia, and Ginger Combination
(*Tang-kuei-szu-ni-chia-wu-shu-yu-sheng-chiang-tang*)
當歸四逆加吳茱萸生薑湯

See page 39.

Uses

Menopausal women with low back pain and abdominal pain due to chilling.

*Pinellia and Magnolia Combination
(*Pan-hsia-hou-pu-tang*) 半夏厚朴湯

See page 91.

Uses

Menopausal anxiety, fear, sorrow, or other strong emotions.

16. Infertility

A woman who wants children but has not been able to conceive over a one year period of unprotected intercourse is said to be barren. Infertility is considered primary (congenital) if she has never conceived and secondary (acquired) if she has been pregnant at least once previously. Absolute or true infertility indicates an incurable causative factor; relative infertility indicates correctible causative factors.

Infertility may originate with either the husband or wife or both. Male infertility results from many factors, such as a lack of viable sperm in the semen, a deformed penis, or impotence. Female infertility also results from a variety of factors, such as nonovulatory menstruation, blocked oviducts, or vaginal and cervical infections. The exact cause or causes can only be determined by a doctor's examination.

Treatment

Some physical causes of infertility cannot be corrected. Others, such as obesity, infection, or consistent failure to have intercourse during the woman's fertile period, are fairly easy to correct. Treatment depends on the specific cause, but Chinese herb formulas may aid conception in women with defective uterine development, chills, or weakness.

Chinese Herbal Formulas

*Tang kuei and Paeonia Formula
(*Tang-kuei-shao-yao-san*) 當歸芍藥散

See page 18.

Uses
Infertility due to defective uterine development, chilling,anemia, and physical weakness.

*Minor Cinnamon and Paeonia Combination
(*Hsiao-chien-chung-tang*) 小建中湯

See page 67.

Uses
Physical weakness, gastrointestinal weakness, and a tendency towards fatigue. For tense abdominal tendons, *tang-kuei* (3.0 gm.) is added.

*Cinnamon and Hoelen Formula
(*Kuei-chih-fu-ling-wan*) 桂枝茯苓丸

See page 15.

Indications
Resistance and pain when pressed on the lower abdomen.

Uses
Infertility due to endometritis, ovaritis, pelviperitonitis, malposition of the uterus, and stagnant blood.

79

*Persica and Rhubarb Combination
(*Tao-ho-cheng-chi-tang*) 桃核承氣湯

See page 16.

Uses
Severe inflammation and congestion in strong patients with constipation.

*Rhubarb and Moutan Combination
(*Ta-huang-mu-tan-pi-tang*) 大黃牡丹皮湯

See page 17.

Indications
Severe resistance and pain when pressed on the lower abdomen, malodorous leukorrhea.

Uses
Strong conformation with pelviperitonitis, cystitis, or stagnant blood.

*Gentiana Combination
(*Lung-tan-hsieh-kan-tang*) 龍膽瀉肝湯

See page 14.

Uses
Strong conformations with infertility due to chronic endometritis, vaginitis, painful urination, or chronic gonorrhea.

*Tang-kuei and Evodia Combination
(Wen-ching-tang) 溫經湯

See page 32.

Uses

Physical weakness, chilling at the waist, hemorrhage, low back pain, diarrhea during menstruation, and a swollen sensation in the lower abdomen.

*Bupleurum and Paeonia Combination
(Chia-wei-hsiao-yao-san) 加味逍遙散

See page 19.

Uses

Infertility due to defects of uterine development or functional disorder of the ovary; hysteria; chlorosis with physical weakness and a tendency towards long-standing anemia.

*Ginseng and Tang-kuei Ten Combination
(Shih-chuan-ta-pu-tang) 十全大補湯

See page 25.

Uses

Severe symptoms of hysteria, chlorosis, anemia, and severe fatigue and weakness in infertile women due to a defective uterus or ovarian disorder.

17. Frigidity

Frigidity usually refers to a woman's habitual lack of pleasure or sexual response during intercourse. Possible causes of frigidity are underdevelopment of the endocrine and nervous systems, immaturity of the male or female genital organs, diseases like diabetes, fear of pregnancy, lack of sexual knowledge, personality conflicts, or unrealistic expectations. Female frigidity does not prevent pregnancy.

Treatment

Physical causes of frigidity require a physician's help. Mental or emotional causes require counseling if serious. Otherwise, openness and understanding between husband and wife and a spirit of cooperation may resolve conflicts or misunderstandings. A little wine or a mild sedative can help the woman relax and reduce emotional tension. The most important point, however, is to identify and resolve the sources of tension or resistance.

Chinese Herbal Formulas

*Bupleurum and Dragon Bone Combination (Chai-hu-chia-lung-ku-mu-li-tang)

柴胡加龍骨牡蠣湯

See page 53.

*Bupleurum and Paeonia Formula
(*Chia-wei-hsiao-yao-san*) 加味逍遙散

See page 19.

Bupleurum Formula
(*I-kan-san*) 抑肝散

Herbal Components

    3.0g *tang-kuei*   3.0g gambir   3.0g cnidium
    4.0g hoelen   2.0g bupleurum 4.0g atractylodes
    1.5g licorice

Gambir is an anti-spasmodic, effective in relieving spasms of the limbs. *Tang-kuei* nourishes hepatic blood. Cnidium improves blood circulation. Bupleurum with licorice and gambir enhance sedative function and alleviate excessive liver *ch'i*. Hoelen and atractylodes are diuretics which can release stagnant water from the stomach.

Uses

    Frigidity due to emotional causes such as nervousness and anxiety.

18. Ovaritis and Oviduct Inflammation

Ovaritis, inflammation of the oviducts (salpingitis), pelviperitonitis, and periovaritis (inflammation around the ovaries) often occur together. The main causes are gonococcus, staphylococcus, and tubercle bacilli or other pathogenic bacteria.

Symptoms of ovaritis are continuous fever, severe pain and fever in the lower abdomen, and occasional yellow pus; chronic ovaritis exhibits ovarian swelling and pain when pressed, continuous pain in the lower abdomen and back, pain during excretion and intercourse, and severe discomfort before the menstrual cycle. Pus, of course, indicates ovarian pustulation. Inflammation of the oviducts causes severe pain in the lower abdomen, a high fever, leukorrhea with pus, difficulty in walking, and spasms in the feet. Severe cases exhibit a continuous fever and can result in peritonitis and become recalcitrant. The condition predisposes a woman toward later tubercular inflammation of the oviducts and ovarian tumors.

Chinese Herbal Formulas

In Chinese medicine, the following formulas are used alone for chronic cases and in conjuction with antibiotics for acute cases.

*Rhubarb and Moutan Combination (*Ta-huang-mu-tan-pi-tang*) 大黃牡丹皮湯

See page 17.

Uses

Acute ovaritis and oviduct inflammation; obvious resistance and pain when pressed on the lower abdomen; polyleukorrhea; severe inflammation.

*Persica and Rhubarb Combination (*Tao-ho-cheng-chi-tang*) 桃核承氣湯

See page 16.

Uses

Acute and subacute resistance and pain when pressed on the lower abdomen, abdominal pain in a strong conformation, severe nervousness, abnormal leukorrhea, and constipation.

*Cinnamon and Hoelen Formula
(*Kuei-chih-fu-ling-wan*) 桂枝茯苓丸

See page 15.

Uses

Chronic symptoms due to moderate inflammation; resistance and pain when pressed on the lower abdomen.

*Gentiana Combination
(*Lung-tan-hsieh-kan-tang*) 龍膽瀉肝湯

See page 14.

Uses

Chronic symptoms, prolonged leukorrhea, and a tense *kan* (liver) meridian on both sides of the umbilicus.

19. Retroflexion of the Uterus

A retroflexed uterus is bent backwards from the normal position. Uterine retroflexion usually presents no problems but causes menstrual aberrations such as excessive menstrual flow, cramps, pain in the lower abdomen and back, and pressure on the bladder and rectum. A retroflexed uterus occasionally causes infertility and may predispose a woman towards endometritis, salpingitis (inflammation of the oviducts), and ovarian ptosis or prolapse (the abnormally low position of an organ). However, simple retroflexion of the uterus usually does not cause the pelvic symptoms listed above.

Treatment

Retroflexion is not treated unless the position of the uterus is definitely causing problems. The condition is determined by insertion of a pessary to hold the uterus in the normal position. If the symptoms disappear and then appear when the pessary is removed because the uterus has returned to a retroflexed position, surgery may be considered.

Chinese Herbal Formulas

Retroflexion may cause stagnant blood. Stagnant blood disrupts blood circulation in the pelvis causing painful and unpleasant intercourse in severe cases. Chinese herb formulas alleviate symptoms of uterine retroflexion.

Tang-kuei and Paeonia Combination (*Tang-kuei-shao-yao-san*) 當歸芍藥散

See page 18.

Uses
Physical weakness, mild anemia, chilling, and a tendency

86

towards fatigue; pain in the lower abdomen and low back pain due to retroversion or retroflexion of the uterus.

*Cinnamon and Hoelen Formula (*Kuei-chih-fu-ling-wan*) 桂枝茯苓丸

See page 15.

Indications
Resistance and pain when pressed on the lower abdomen.

Uses
Retroflexion of the uterus, endometritis or oviduct inflammation, stagnant blood. When there is constipation, rhubarb (0.5-2.0g) is added.

*Persica and Rhubarb Combination (*Tao-ho-cheng-chi-tang*) 桃核承氣湯

See page 16.

Uses
Severe cases of inflammation, ruddy face, congestion, and headache.

*Tang-kuei and Evodia Combination (*Wen-ching-tang*) 溫經湯

See page 32.

Uses
Chilling, infertility due to retroflexion of the uterus,

difficult menstruation, pain in the lower abdomen, hot palms and dry lips.

*Bupleurum and Paeonia Formula (*Chia-wei-hsiao-yao-san*) 加味逍遙散

See page 19.

Uses

Abdominal swelling, anemia, and nervousness. Addition of 3.0g each of rehmannia and cyperus will enhance the results.

20. Prolapse of the Uterus

A uterine prolapse exists when the uterus has fallen backwards and downwards into the vagina, either partially or completely. The usual cause of prolapse is failure for whatever reason of the surrounding ligaments to support the uterus in its normal position.

Treatment

Surgery. In women who are poor risks, a pessary can hold the uterus in position.

Chinese Herbal Formulas

Chinese herb formulas improve the constitution for surgery if necessary or dispel the pressure of stagnant blood in the abdomen which is often present in cases of prolapse.

*Tang-kuei and Paeonia Formula
(*Tang-kuei-shao-yao-san*) 當歸芍藥散

See page 18.

Uses
Chills, mild anemia, and physical weakness.

*Cinnamon and Hoelen Formula
(*Kuei-chih-fu-ling-wan*) 桂枝茯苓丸

See page 15.

Uses
Rather strong conformations with stagnant blood in the lower abdomen and pressure from a tumor. If there is constipation and severe stagnant blood, Persica and Rhubarb Combination is recommended instead.

*Ginseng and Astragalus Combination
(*Pu-chung-i-chi-tang*) 補中益氣湯

First prescribed by Li Tung-yuan, one of the great physicians of the thirteenth century. It is known as the "king of all prescriptions" and is widely used to increase vigor and body strength.

Herbal Components
    4.0g astragalus   2.0g citrus   2.0g bupleurum
    4.0g ginseng   3.0g *tang-kuei*   2.0g ginger

1.5g licorice   1.0g cimicifuga   2.0g jujube
4.0g atractylodes

Ginseng and astragalus nourish the lungs and act as antihidrotics (agents which inhibit sweating). Ginseng and licorice nourish the spleen and the stomach as well as increasing vitality. *Tang-kuei* nourishes the blood and in combination with astragalus nourishes the skin. Atractylodes and citrus improve the functioning of the spleen and stomach. Bupleurum and cimicifuga are antipyretics (agents which reduce or prevent fever). Ginger and jujube coordinate the actions of the other herbs.

Indications
Weak pulse, general fatigue, mild fever, headache, night sweats, hypotension, hemorrhoids, loss of appetite.

Uses
Physical weakness and anemia. The formula is often combined with kaolin (3.0 gm.).

Tang-kuei and Evodia Combination
(*Wen-ching-tang*) 溫經湯

See page 32.

Uses
Uterine ptosis in weak women with menstrual aberration, waist chills and abdominal pain, congestion, chilling, dry lips, and hot palms.

Tang-kuei, Evodia, and Ginger Combination
(*Tang-kuei-szu-ni-chia-wu-chu-yu-sheng-chiang-tang*)
當歸四逆加吳茱萸生薑湯

See page 39.

Uses
Severe chills, a tendency towards anemia, abdominal pain when the patient feels cold, severe ptosis.

*Coptis and Scute Combination
(*Huang-lien-chieh-tu-tang*) 黃連解毒湯

See page 63.

Uses
Moderate symptoms.

*Pinellia and Magnolia Combination
(*Pan-hsia-hou-pu-tang*) 半夏厚朴湯

First mentioned in the Chinese medical work *Summaries of Household Remedies* (Chin kuei yao lueh) of the Han dynasty.

Herbal Components
6.0g pinellia   5.0g hoelen   4.0g ginger
3.0g magnolia bark   2.0g perilla
Pinellia and hoelen relieve fluid accumulation, alleviate nausea and vomiting, and increase blood circulation. Magnolia bark treats abdominal fullness and increases vitality. Perilla has a tranquilizing effect and increases gastrointestinal function. Ginger acts as a diuretic, alleviates vomiting, increases gastrointestinal function, and coordinates the action of the other herbs.

Uses
Weak patients who have a sensation of something blocking or itching and stimulating the throat, a hoarse

voice, weak and sunken pulse, and a patting sound at the lower part of the heart.

21. Skin Problems

In cultures where marriage is one of the few life-supporting alternatives available to women, the condition of the skin is of prime importance to them, and it is in this context that Chinese medicine places skin disorders under gynecology. A case in point is acne, usually a phenomenon of youth. In a male, acne is regarded as a natural part of growing up. Contrarily, a female with this problem, especially after she has become eligible for marriage, is thought to be extremely unattractive and socially unacceptable. The aura surrounding acne is not as harsh in the Western cultures. Nonetheless, there are more girls than boys suffering from the physical and pyschological consequences of acne, no doubt due to the complex hormonal systems of women. Even while acne does not threaten one's life, it has extremely unpleasant effects on women, particularly in their social lives.

Cosmetics preserve and restore beauty. Yet in spite of the profusion of cosmetic products available, many people have ugly skin and skin disorders. It stands to reason that proper skin care cannot solely depend upon cosmetics which are topical. Skin condition is inextricably linked to internal factors as well as external ones. The skin reflects diet and lifestyle, or as is said in China, the skin mirrors the viscera. Formulas for skin problems mainly nourish the viscera and improve the constitution.

Acne

Acne results from disturbances in the sebaceous glands that cause excessive sebum to block the pores of the skin. Infection and consequent suppuration are usually due to pyogenic cocci. Western medicine links *acne vulgaris* of adolescence to an imbalance of androgen and estrogen, the hormones secreted by the sexual glands. Those individuals with oily skin are highly susceptible. Gastrointestinal disturbances, liver disorders, hormonal disorders, and constipation are secondary causes. For unknown reasons, the condition aggravates just before each menstrual period.

Western medicine has yet to effectively treat acne, but neither has Chinese medicine achieved unqualified success. The Chinese formulas which treat the condition revitalize the sufferer's constitution. Since ugly skin corresponds directly to such internal factors as dietary and hormonal imbalances, certain Chinese herbal formulas specifically adjust or regulate the female hormones.

Chinese Herbal Formulas

Tang-kuei and Paeonia Formula
(*Tang-kuei-shao-yao-san*) 當歸芍藥散

See page 18.

Uses

Acne; coarse skin and blemishes. Contraindicated for those with a robust physique and *nobose* (a spontaneous flushing sensation). If the formula nauseates the patient, a third of a dosage of Cardamon and Fennel Formula (*An-chung-san*) may be taken.

93

Coarse Skin on the Hands

The Japanese call this condition "goosefoot wind" (*eh-yen-fang*) because the skin becomes dry and coarse like a goose's foot. In modern medical terms it is known as sudamen. Characterized by noninflammatory eruptions of whitish vesicles caused by the retention of sweat in the corneous layer of the skin, it is found in women more often than in men. Sometimes the finger whorls cannot be seen or are torn and painful. Sudamen often results from the use of laundry detergents and chemical cleaning agents. However, the basic etiology seems to be linked to hormonal disorders, to the autonomic nervous system, or to the heart. The real cause is still unknown and modern medicine finds the condition resistant to treatment.

Coarse skin can also be caused by frigorism, a condition resulting from long exposure to the cold. When the skin is exposed to cold air, the blood vessels contract, the blood condenses, and numbness sets in. Those most susceptible to frigorism are those with chilblains and those who fail to take proper care of themselves.

Chinese Herbal Formulas

Tang-kuei, Evodia, and Ginger Combination (*Tang-kuei-szu-ni-chia-wu-chu-yu-sheng-chiang-tang*)
當歸四逆加吳茱萸生薑湯

See page 39.

Uses

Coarse skin caused by frigorism.

94

Bupleurum and Paeonia Formula
(*Chia-wei-hsiao-yao-san*) 加味逍遙散

See page 19.

Uses
    Sudamen or coarse skin.

Cinnamon and Hoelen Formula
(*Kuei-chih-fu-ling-wan*) 桂枝茯苓丸

See page 15.

Uses
    Sudamen or coarse skin.

Tang-kuei and Paeonia Formula
(*Tang-kuei-shao-yao-san*) 當歸芍藥散

See page 18.

Uses
    Sudamen or coarse skin.

Atractylodes Combination
(*Yueh-pi-chia-chu-tang*) 越婢加朮湯

Herbal Components
    6.0g *ma-huang*   2.0g licorice   8.0g gypsum
    3.0g jujube   3.0g ginger   4.0g atractylodes

Uses
Sudamen in a strong conformation with dry throat and infrequent urination.

Tang-kuei and Gardenia Combination
(*Wen-ching-yin*) 溫清飲

Herbal Components
4.0g *tang-kuei*	4.0g cnidium	1.5g phellodendron
4.0g rehmannia	1.5g coptis	2.0g gardenia
4.0g paeonia	3.0g scute	

Indications
Menstrual aberrations and irregularity, pain at the waist, cold extremities, feverish palms, aching hands.

Uses
Eczema and skin diseases such as sudamen in a weak conformation with bleeding, uterine bleeding, and anemia.

Pityriasis Versicolor

A mild, chronic, fungal infection of the superficial layer of the skin characterized by scaly discolored areas. Pityriasis versicolor is of two types. The first, a local infection, usually occurs in people fifty or older. The second, characterized by spotty white discoloration of the skin due to a deficiency of skin pigment, usually occurs in the middle-aged. The white patches gradually extend. As they reach an area of hair growth, the hair turns white. There are no other obvious symptoms. Intestinal diseases accompanied by fever, scarlet fever, neurosis, sensitivity to external medications, injury, and continuous stress are thought to cause this lack of pigmentation. Some think it is caused by malnutrition or a disorder of the autonomic nervous system. The true causes, however, have not been clearly established. It is not amenable to treatment with Western medicine.

Chinese Herbal Formulas

Cinnamon and Astragalus Combination
(*Kuei-chih-chia-huang-chi-tang*) 桂枝加黃耆湯

Herbal Components
4.0g cinnamon   4.0g ginger   4.0g paeonia
3.0g astragalus   4.0g jujube

Indications
Pityriasis versicolor.

Uses
Persons prone to skin diseases and infections who perspire easily.

Bupleurum and Paeonia Formula
(*Chia-wei-hsiao-yao-san*) 加味逍遙散

See page 19.

Uses
Pityriasis in the presence of anemia, menstrual disorders, or nervous disorders.

Cinnamon and Hoelen Formula plus Coix (6 g)
(*Kuei-chih-fu-ling-wan-chia-i-yi-jen*)
桂枝茯苓丸加薏苡仁

See page 15.

Uses

Pityriasis accompanied with stagnant blood.

Body Odor

In a woman, odors usually originate in the vaginal area and the armpits. Chinese medicine attributes a propensity toward malodorous sweating to water toxin. Usually the patient herself is unaware of the odor but others find it quite offensive. Body odor ensues after the onset of hormonal activity at puberty. When a person reaches an advanced age the odor usually disappears.

Chinese Herbal Formulas

Stephania and Astragalus Combination (*Fang-chi-huang-chi-tang*) 防己黃耆湯

See page 72.

Uses

Body odors.

*Gentiana Combination (*Lung-tang-hsieh-kan-tang*) 龍膽瀉肝湯

See page 16.

Uses

Body odors.

Note: The page number which appears first locates the primary information about each herbal formula. Page numbers are not always in consecutive order.

Index

A

B

H

L

M

P

References

Hsu, Hong-yen   How to Treat Yourself with Chinese Herbs
               Los Angeles: Oriental Healing Arts Ins-
               titute, 1980

Hsu, Hong-yen and Hsu, Chau-shin   Commonly Used Chinese
               Herb Formulas with Illustrations
               Los Angeles: Oriental Healing Arts Ins-
               titute, 1980

Hsu, Hong-yen and Peacher, William C.   Chinese Herb
               Medicine and Therapy
               Los Angeles: Oriental Healing Arts Ins-
               titute, 1982

Nishiyama, Hideo   Kanpo igaku no kiso do shinryo (漢方医学
               の基礎と診療 Fundamentals of Kanpo and
               Therapy)
               Osaka: Sogensha, 1969

————————————   Josei do kanpo (女性と漢方 Women and Kanpo)
               Osaka: Sogensha, 1975

About the Authors

Dr. Hong-yen Hsu has a distinguished background in research and teaching. After graduation from the Meiji Pharmaceutical College and the Pharmacognosy Department of Tokyo University, Dr. Hsu earned his Doctor of Pharmacy degree at the University of Kyoto. He remained in Japan for three more years as a member of the research staff of the Department of Pharmaceutical Science at the University of Tokyo before returning to Taiwan in 1945. Since that time he has been actively engaged in teaching and conducting research at National Taiwan University and the medical colleges at Taipei, Taichung, and Kaohsiung. He has also served as acting chief of the Taiwan Provincial Hygienic Laboratory and as the director of the Food and Drug Control Bureau of the National Health Administration. Currently Dr. Hsu is a professor in the Botany Department at the Chinese Culture University and the Institute of Pharmacological Science at the China Medical College, and president of the Brion Research Institute of Taiwan. Dr. Hsu's foresight led to the founding of the Oriental Healing Arts Institute in 1976. The institute is dedicated to furthering research and understanding of Chinese traditional medicine. A prolific author, he has published more than one hundred articles and books.

Douglas Easer is director of public relations and a research associate at the Oriental Healing Arts Institute. He is a Ph.D. candidate in Chinese History at the University of Kansas.

DATE DUE

OCT 1 1 1998			
OCT 2 6 1999			
NO 19 '99			